Smell

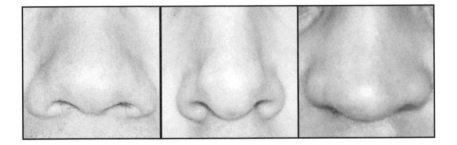

The Secret Seducer

Translated from the Dutch by Paul Vincent

Smell

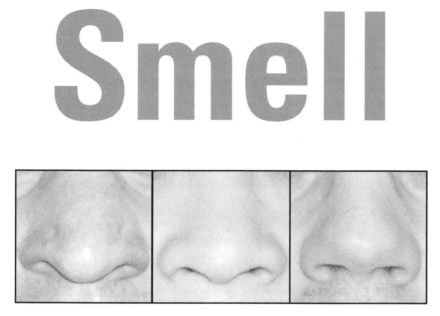

Piet Vroon

with Anton van Amerongen and Hans de Vries

Farrar, Straus and Giroux • New York

Farrar, Straus and Giroux
19 Union Square West, New York 10003

Distributed in Canada by Douglas & McIntyre Ltd.
Printed in the United States of America

Designed by Abby Kagan
Nose photographs by Mark Maguire (left to right): Jonathan Lippincott,
Mark Maguire, Audrey Gillespie-Jobson, Peter Buchanan-Smith, Eleen Chung,
Peter Richardson

First published in Dutch in 1994 under the title *Verborgen verleider* by
Uitgeverij AMBO, Baarn
First Farrar, Straus and Giroux edition, 1997

Library of Congress Cataloging-in-Publication Data
Vroon, P. A.
    [Verborgen verleider.   English]
    Smell : the secret seducer / Piet Vroon ; with Anton van Amerongen
and Hans de Vries ; translated from the Dutch by Paul Vincent.
        p.   cm.
    Includes bibliographical references.
    ISBN 0-374-25704-3 (alk. paper)
    1. Smell—Physiological aspects.   2. Smell—Psychological aspects.
I. Amerongen, Anton van, 1959-   . II. Vries, Hans de, 1949-
III. Title.
QP458.V757   1997
612.8'6—DC21   97-2299

Contents

Foreword

This book is a co-production and came into existence by chance, to the extent that three people who are intrigued by the strange sense of smell embarked on a joint enterprise. Piet Vroon is a professor of psychology at the University of Utrecht in the Netherlands; his original psychological work was in the field of olfactory research. Anton van Amerongen is a biologist, and Hans de Vries is an independent psychologist; he has concentrated on the language and readability of the text. Briefly summarized, the following topics are dealt with.

Chapter 1 discusses the cultural and scientific history of smell, including some facts about smell in the animal kingdom.

Chapter 2 focuses on the structure and operation of the olfactory organ, and the way olfactory sensations originate. This account includes some rather technical biological passages; readers with no interest in this information can skip or skim a few sections. It is, however, necessary to acquaint oneself with a number of concepts for a full understanding of the rest of the book.

Chapter 3 deals with the "psychophysics" of smell. What is the link between the intensity of a stimulus and the ensuing perception? How does conditioning to smells take place? In what way can odors reinforce or inhibit one another? And what can this information tell us about how to combat smell pollution?

Chapter 4 discusses both interpersonal differences in the field of olfactory capacity and the appreciation of smells, and differences that occur in a single person. What changes does our sense of smell undergo in our lifetime? To what extent is the perception of smells dependent on sex, age, lifestyle, occupation, culture and the like?

Smells are not only perceived but also remembered and described in words. To what extent can we do this? Do blind people smell better than people with all their senses intact? Do perfumers perform better in smell tests than other people? These and similar questions are dealt with in Chapter 5.

Smells have considerable influence on our behavior and even on our bodily functioning. Examples are the regulation of mood and general activity, sex and motivation, and the way in which we judge each other in all kinds of situations (Chapter 6).

For some reason many people stock up with artificial odors in the form of perfumes and lotions; apart from that each of us has a so-called olfactory passport or personal "aroma"—a body or breath odor family members and others can recognize (Chapter 7).

Chapter 8 deals with olfactory disorders, and the link between smell and disease. The book concludes with a number of tips and recommendations.

P.V.
A.v.A.
H.d.V.
Fall 1994

Smell is the sense of memory and desire.

—Rousseau

Smell

Chapter 1

The History of Smelling

The nose is centrally located on the human face; it is a perennial in fashion and cosmetics, and indispensable for those of us who wear eyeglasses. In social and cultural life and literature, too, the nose is a familiar feature—one need look no further than the many proverbs, sayings, nicknames, and terms of abuse that relate to this striking part of the face.

The nose also forms the external section of the olfactory organ, however, and as such it does not receive the attention it deserves. For example, too few people are aware that breathing through the nose is vital to both physical and mental health. This method of breathing ensures that the air is to some extent warmed and filtered, and in addition it creates the correct pressure in the arteries in the chest cavity.[1] Finally, one smells more when one breathes through the nose, which generally benefits mood and memory.

The Importance of Smell

Taste and smell together are the so-called chemical senses, meaning that stimuli associated with them are chemically based. In many respects the sense of smell is mysterious—not only because little is known about its operation as yet, but also because most people are insufficiently aware of its importance. When people are asked what sense they would be prepared to do without if necessary, smell comes at the top of the list and sight at the bottom. This is a debatable choice, given that smell plays a significant part in many psychic processes and behavior patterns. Smell is essential for the operation of the sense of taste; it affects one's sex life, motivation and memory processes (including learning, health and feelings of security and well-being); and it has an alarm function in life-threatening situations (for instance, in detecting gas fumes, etc.). What is more, in "competition" (that is, when several senses are stimulated simultaneously), the nose often comes out on top. A beautiful-looking apple that smells rotten does not whet our appetite.

A Brief Cultural History

Historically, the debate over the status of smell has been a complicated one; in Western countries in particular, thinking on this sense has had a decidedly ambiguous quality.[2] Plato denounced perfumes because they played into the hands of effeminacy and physical pleasure; the use of aromatics was reserved for prostitutes. In his view the virtuous should be concerned mainly with cultivating the good of their souls through music and mathematics. The body with all its odors was only the temporary tomb of the soul; moreover, because of its position close to the brain, the nose was in direct contact with feelings and desires that were better banished. Socrates was somewhat less dogmatic in this matter: he felt that odors reflected the social class to which a person belonged, meaning that an odor had a certain informative value.[3]

In general, though, Plato regarded the eye and the ear as more important aids than the nose. In social intercourse, hearing and particularly sight are "noble" activities, he believed, because those senses bring us into contact with the world of perfection. Geometry is discovered through sight; the Pythagoreans' music of the spheres is "heard"; taste is already somewhat ambiguous, and many philosophers considered touching and smelling vulgar and often rather sordid activities.[4] Man walks upright—so went another common line of reasoning, also put forward by Freud—which means that with the aid of his faculty of sight man can see what is happening around him from a long way off. Unlike animals, it was claimed, we scarcely need smell, any more than we need a tail. The idea is not absurd. Many odors are heavier than air, so that one smells more when lying on the ground than when standing.

Later philosophers wrote scarcely anything about smell, and if they did (one example is Kant at the end of the eighteenth century), they generally disparaged this sense. Partly as a result, virtually no research was carried out into the operation of the sense of smell, while a great deal of attention was paid to the sense of sight.

During the "scientific revolution," the Enlightenment and the Industrial Revolution, great emphasis was placed on the intellect. Human rationality was seen as *the* engine of progress. This meant that a certain contempt arose for emotions and for the body as a whole. That also applied to smell, since that sense is associated with (unpleasant) bodily and breath odors among other things—a view that was in the tradition of both Plato and Kant.

On the other hand, with regard to smell and the importance of the senses in general, a part was also played by English empiricism, which located the source of all knowledge in the senses. Given the idea that knowledge was based entirely on experience, many scientific researchers (and the doctors and chemists who collaborated with them) started using their senses, including smell, in a more intensive way. It is remarkable that it took so long to discover a link between smells and chemical substances. The renowned Dutch physician Boerhaave, for example, still believed that an odor was based on a separate "fluidum," called *spiritus rector*, which was supposed to be oily in character.[5] The same applied to the air: chemists did not know initially that air consists of a mixture of elements and compounds.

However, the major impulse which led to the increasing attention paid to smell, particularly in the eighteenth and early nineteenth centuries, came from medicine. Because of a lack of understanding of the nature and origin of (infectious) diseases, doctors and researchers sought the cause of all kinds of ailments and epidemics, including plague and malaria (literally "bad air"), in noxious vapors (*miasmas*) released from rotting corpses, urine and feces, swamps, vapors that rose from cracks after earthquakes (according to the *physica subterranea*, the bowels of the earth contained a quite dangerous "stench laboratory," capable of making mankind sick), down to the feather bed or "a veritable hodgepodge of mephitic exhalations," as someone wrote (*mephitic* means both stinking and poisonous). Those miasmas were commonly found in hospitals and prisons, where not only many inmates but also many lawyers were supposed to have died as a result of the stench. As late as the nineteenth century judges visiting prisons tried to protect themselves against typhus by surrounding themselves with "antimephitic" odors.[6]

One doctor of the period observed that the smell of his flatulence was virtually indistinguishable from the smell of the cadavers in the dissecting room. The processes of decomposition in the intestines and the principle of life were a unity within a living organism, he surmised, but the other side of the coin was that noxious odors were also absorbed through the skin. It was even conceivable that breathing in the last gasp of a dying person through one's nose might prove fatal, because the deadly poison rushed to the brain.[7] One must also be careful about inhaling the breath of cattle; this might result in attacks of colic and nausea. (Garlic was used until late in the nineteenth century to ward off evil spirits.) Doctors preferred to examine the patient with one hand, while with the other they held under their nose boxes filled with amber, sulphur and a kind of incense. Next of kin and others interested in visiting the sick were instructed to dress in thick clothes and told not to swallow their saliva but to spit it out.

This line of thinking led to a frantic hunt for "antimephitic remedies," which could eliminate both the stench and the danger of disease, a hunt that eventually led to the lighting of fires, to which a purifying action was ascribed, and only much later to the discovery of disinfectants such as bleach (1788). Some chemists went so far as to gird themselves with jars in order to collect their bodily odors for closer analysis; an Italian canon hired beggars for this purpose, enclosing them in leather bags up to their waists.

At the time, puerperal fever was attributed to the atmosphere and not to hands infected with microorganisms. As a result, the Hungarian doctor Semmelweis was ridiculed when in 1847 he claimed that puerperal fever could be prevented if doctors and obstetricians washed their hands before each treatment (the delivery room was close to the mortuary). Semmelweis believed that an "infectious substance" deriving from the mortuary caused this serious illness. Despite the fact that when hand washing was practiced the death rate among mothers in childbirth fell by 90 percent, there was such violent opposition to this idea that Semmelweis was forced to leave Vienna. Only after several decades (and many hundreds of unnecessary deaths) were his ideas accepted.

Because odors were supposed to reveal what was happening in the body, an extensive system of diagnosis was developed on the basis of the smells of sweat, breath and blood, as well as urine, stools, sputum, ulcers, pus and even the gaps between toes and under the armpits (the foundation for these practices was laid in the eleventh century by the Arab physician Avicenna). And as far as medical instruments were concerned: the stethoscope did not come into general use because it enabled the doctor to hear what was going on in the body better; rather, it permitted the doctor to avoid unnecessary contact with stench. Conversely, doctors used scents in therapy (aromatherapy, osmotherapy, herbal baths). Particularly volatile, warm, oily and aromatic substances as well as "air cures" in the mountains were supposed to ensure that the "vital spirits" started flowing properly again through the (hypothetical) tubes in the body.[8]

Since bodily and breath odors were regarded as deriving from habits of life and the quality of vital juices, there were powerful pronouncements in other areas too. It was claimed that women's bodily fluids could be spoiled through excessive sexual intercourse (through too much semen, that is). Because of this prostitutes were referred to as *les putains*, "the stinking ones" (a term used in antiquity by the poet Juvenal). Homosexuals also had a hard time of it. These people were often found in the vicinity of public latrines, and the animal stench that surrounded them was taken to represent their "anality." Another view held by doctors in the past was that sperm stimulates the organs and fibers of the body; the seed produces the stench given off by strong men, which eunuchs are deprived of. The bodily and breath odors of the virile man were (therefore) called the *aura seminalis*. Rage was supposed to heighten a man's bodily smell even further, as it accelerated the breakdown of gall. Such notions led many experts to advise men not to wash: this might cause them to lose their sexual attraction. For their part, women's aura was permeated with milk: "Our women sweat milk, urinate milk, chew and pass milk when they blow their noses, and excrete milk with their stools," wrote one doctor in a manual on chronic diseases.

Because of the fear of disease and epidemics, the unimaginable stench that prevailed almost everywhere led to interventions by "hygienists" and municipal health boards. The hygienists succeeded in combating the stench in cities, hospitals, prisons and private dwellings. Closed sewage systems were constructed, ventilators and bellows positioned, factories shut down, hospitals equipped with commodes and chamber pots, churchyards treated with salt, lime and sulphuric acid, cesspits emptied, codes of conduct for sewage workers drawn up, stinking marshes drained, walls, vaults and woodwork plastered, filled, painted and whitewashed to combat miasmas; even furniture was treated with antimephitic varnish. One Scottish hygienist went so far as to smash the windows of workers' homes in order to let loose the stench.

As in Plato's time, the predominantly negative significance given to smell and all kinds of odors led many scholars to assign this sense a place at the bottom of the hierarchy of senses: "as the sense of lust, desire and impulse it carries the stamp of animality," as someone wrote. Most smells were to be *gotten rid of*.

Apart from the medical perspective, the association of smell with animality was also justified in the following terms: animals sniff a lot and, moreover, man is often not capable of expressing smells in language, a capacity which is quintessentially human and testifies to civilization. Therefore smell was supposed to have more animal than human traits. We still find traces of this view in the value attached to certain occupations. Those who deal with stench tend to be low on the social ladder: the sewage worker, the toilet lady, the garbageman, the farmhand.

Against the background of these views the washing of the human body led to heated disputes. One school of thought held that if you kept yourself dirty you could prevent miasmas from penetrating your unprotected skin; moreover, your body would be weakened by frequent contact with water. What's more, if you bathed too often you were running the risk of becoming sexually unattractive; you might even end up infertile. Others believed, however, that you could rid your body of sickly exhalations by cleaning your skin, as a result of which many bathing regulations were drawn up.[9] You should clean at least the visible parts of your body, such experts believed, with the ideal being the mother-of-pearl skin in which you could see the blue blood coursing through your veins. A translucent body was the mirror of a pure soul; at the same time, this sort of washing was a way to curb women's passions. Bathing was useful for restraining sexual urges, as one Father Marie de Saint Ursin proclaimed at the beginning of the nineteenth century: "If a pale girl . . . seeks out solitude and gives herself over to melancholy fantasies, then a prolonged hot bath may moderate the causes of this erotic orgasm." (Victims of passion were also advised to lead a sedentary life, stay in the shade, and wear gloves to protect their hands.) After bathing—a ritual which must certainly not be performed more than once a week —the woman must keep her eyes closed when drying her genitalia, and young girls were advised to stir up the water to prevent the surface from becoming a mirror when they got into the bath. After the "second shiver," the unfortunate persons rested from their exertions.

Not all scientific researchers, philosophers and artists stressed rationality to the extent that the Enlightenment philosophers did. Rousseau and Goethe recognized the great importance of intuition and emotional involvement, in the pursuit of science too, and even praised the sense of smell. Indeed, in the *Romantic* period, such concepts as *Sturm und Drang* and *Weltschmerz*, and artistic expressions like Novalis's *Hymnen an die Nacht* and the nocturnes of Chopin, attached great importance to feelings and emotional life in general, including unpleasant smells. The Romantics tried to overcome the limitations of bourgeois existence by living in seclusion, plumbing their feelings, seeking intoxication (by using stimulants, etc.) and losing themselves in melancholy (the *paradis artificiels* we find in Baudelaire). Eroticism, too, regained some esteem as a vital part of life.[10]

Apart from these philosophical considerations, there was a simple yet universal change in the attitude toward the sense of smell: because of developments in chemistry and (later) bacteriology, doctors began using their noses much less. However, the conviction that stench does not normally contain germs dates only from about 1880. And while the Romantics glorified sensual happiness, including smell, not everyone agreed. The sense of smell was still primarily associated with sex; both were considered reprehensible in many Western cultures, again because of their age-old associations with animality. By Freud's time smell had emerged again (temporarily) at least in the literature, albeit negatively (in Freud's view smell was most closely linked with feces and with the "anal phase" of psychological development).

Another influential figure was Freud's contemporary and associate W. Fliess, the ear, nose and throat specialist. Fliess developed a comprehensive "nose theory" of sexuality, claiming, for example, that there was a "reflex neurosis," based on connections between smell and the genitals. Fliess performed minor operations on the inside of the nose in order to alleviate psychic and gynecological ailments. The administering of cocaine was also part of his therapeutic arsenal.[11]

At this time "animal" smells like leather and musk were regarded as aphrodisiacs. Here is Zola, the Naturalist par excellence: "With the aid of a piece of musk she abandons herself to forbidden delights. She is in the habit of surreptitiously sniffing it. She drugs herself with it until orgiastic convulsions overwhelm her." And Balzac: "In the boarding school the mephitism of the walls, the stench of the staff and the semen smell of the invigilator and the masturbating pupils mounted. This stench, experienced as typically male, heightens the desire for the presence of women." "Shit in the boots, piss out of the window, cry shit, have a good crap, fart loudly, smoke like a chimney, belch in people's faces," Flaubert advised a friend.[12] During Queen Victoria's state visit to France in 1855, there was an outcry at court, where the sensitive noses of the ladies thought they detected her wearing perfume containing a little musk.

In short, Western cultures have had a love-hate relationship with the sense of smell. And if we look at the war waged nowadays in the commercials over sanitary pads, tampons, diapers for infants and adults, sweet-smelling soaps, skin-care products, deodorants, perfumes and the like, we can say that smell is considered important once again.

It is striking that history seems to be repeating itself to some extent. Just as in the past the atmosphere and odors were blamed for countless evils on the basis of almost hysterical prejudices, something similar is happening today with those who are HIV-positive and AIDS patients. In the view of many celebrated researchers, including the discoverer of the virus, L. Montagnier, it is not certain that the HIV virus alone is a sufficient precondition for the devastation of the human immune system (he claims that much more would be needed); moreover, one must receive a substantial amount of the virus directly or indirectly in one's blood. Nevertheless, many people believe that it is better not to touch people who are HIV-positive, to avoid contact with their clothes even, and by all means to keep from kissing them. Since there is no indication of any risk whatsoever in such actions, an obvious analogy presents itself with the absurd advice about avoiding smells given to those visiting the sick centuries ago.

Smell and Science

The scientific world is still not very much interested in the olfactory organ: the number of researchers worldwide is a few hundred at most. There are various possible explanations for this.

Scents and associated olfactory sensations are not nearly as easy to measure or map as stimuli and observations based on light and sound: after all, a scent has no wavelength or other easily measurable property. Moreover, olfactory sensations are triggered by chemical substances of very different kinds, which are difficult to group under a single common denominator. Our knowledge of the operation of the sense of smell is so poor that we do not know exactly what properties of chemical substances cause the sensations. Strictly speaking, we don't even know whether chemical characteristics of substances are responsible for olfactory sensations, or whether, to mention just one possibility, the *shape* of the molecule is responsible (the key-lock principle or the so-called stereochemical theory).[13] A researcher has expressed this uncertainty as follows: "It is still impossible to predict with any degree of accuracy whether a chemical compound will have a smell, and if so, what qualitative properties that smell will have."[14] That is no small admission, certainly compared with our knowledge of other senses.

Olfactory research also has many technical problems to contend with. Odors can interact with their environment in all kinds of ways before we perceive them. This means that the experimental area and the equipment used must be odor-free, and that the researcher must be very familiar with the doses used. Only in the second half of the twentieth century have researchers developed good "olfactometers"—apparatus for administering carefully calculated quantities of odors.

Research is further complicated by the fact that people display wide differences both in their sensitivity to smells and in their appreciation of smells. All kinds of diseases or congenital defects may underlie these differences, but even among normal, healthy people the sense of smell varies enormously. Two extremes are general *anosmia*, an inability to smell, and *hyperosmia*, an oversensitivity to olfactory stimuli. Moreover, depending on the circumstances there is also a great deal of variation within the same individual: one processes the smell of fried eggs differently the morning after a drinking binge than on the evening of the same day after a healthy ramble through the woods. "There are days when I am moved by the slightest smell; on others, far more numerous, I smell nothing," Maine de Biran wrote in 1815, noting the favorable days, like May 13 of that year, when "the wonderfully perfumed air that I breathe in makes me glad to be alive."[15]

In general, women have a keener sense of smell than men, and older people regain their olfactory capacity less quickly than younger people after an "olfactory bombardment." The range of smells on offer also varies from country to country and village to village. As a result, it is possible for people to lose their ability to distinguish certain smells to a greater or lesser extent through conditioning; members of a particular culture, for example, may develop extreme sensitivity to certain (say, dangerous) smells.

Finally, the world of smells is difficult to pin down in concrete terms. The available vocabulary for describing smells is very limited. Often smells are simply related back to their supposed source. "This smells of coffee" or "It smells like after a thunderstorm in August here." The results of a recent experiment demonstrate this relative inability: different respondents described the smell of isobutyraldehyde as that of "chocolate," "peanut butter sandwich," "sickly and dry," "sour milk," "codfish," "endives" or "cocoa"; strikingly, a third of those involved could not describe the smell in any terms at all.[16]

This phenomenon can be understood partly on the basis of evolution. In evolutionary terms the sense of smell is an old one, with relatively few direct connections with the youngest part of the brain—namely, the left neocortex, a system which houses, for example, "language centers." It does have many well-developed connections with older brain structures that regulate emotions and motivation, including the so-called limbic system, the brain stem or the "neural chassis," together with the "president" of the hormonal system, the hypophysis or pituitary gland. Via the pituitary gland, smell influences general bodily function (hormone production). One result of this construction is that we do not in the first instance rationalize and verbalize what we smell, but have an immediate *reaction* to a smell and a tendency to act in accordance with it. In other words, people do not generally convert an olfactory perception into a considered intellectual judgment followed by consciously controlled behavior; smelling something generally leads to emotionally colored and sometimes even instinctive actions.

The commercial interests of the cosmetics and food industries play important parts in olfactory research, and olfactory researchers generally profit from government and industrial support. Over and against this support (and perhaps because of it), no research of importance has been carried out into topics like olfactory disorders, which often have serious consequences (such as memory problems and depressions), or into substances that may affect our moods, performance and possibly diseases. For example, there are indications that Alzheimer's disease originates with a decline in the olfactory capacity, a process which might be preventable.

It is both reprehensible and strange that so little attention is paid to the way in which smells (apart from perfumes) can affect our behavior, our social interaction and our well-being. After all, everybody knows that factors such as excessive noise, poor ventilation and the color or temperature of artificial lighting affect our well-being, so why is there almost no research into how we are affected by smells?

Senses in the Animal Kingdom

An efficient supply of information is of great importance to every living organism. The scope for experimentation in nature is limited; the various animal species consequently have reasonably comparable sets of tools. There is a fair degree of similarity in eyes, noses, taste buds and organs of touch and balance. One species, though, may sometimes have a specific aid. For example, bees can detect the direction of polarization of sunlight, and rattlesnakes have infrared detectors close to their eyes, with the aid of which they can find prey through temperature registration.

The sensitivity and range of these senses, however, vary enormously from species to species. The mole is virtually blind, but potentially it has the same kind of eye as the eagle. For that matter, the eagle can see virtually nothing at a short distance; the bird is extremely farsighted. Cats have a mirroring or reflective layer of cells behind their retina (*tunica luminosa*), as a result of which the light passes through their sensory cells twice. Consequently, cats have excellent vision in twilight, but during the day their world is virtually colorless. Moreover, the perception of colors may be based on two pigments in the retina (in dichromates), but also on three, four or even five pigments (in pentachromates, such as pigeons). Animals in the pentachromate group can distinguish colors and shades of color that we cannot even imagine.

Quails are stone deaf, like most fishes, although a number of freshwater species can hear reasonably well (and taste and smell, too). Bats "see" with their ears. They emit high-pitched sounds, the echo of which enables them to locate objects. The system is so precise that the bat is able to pinpoint and catch moths with it. On the other hand, many species of moths have developed ears that are sensitive to the frequencies emitted by the bat. These moths will drop straight to the ground when they hear the sound, thus eluding the bat's "radar," as it were.

The more important the role gravity plays in the life of an animal, the more important it is for the creature to be able to keep its balance. The cat traditionally lands on its feet, and you need have no qualms about throwing a spider off a tower; at worst, the creature will sustain some minor bruises. Balance also helps an animal to navigate efficiently. The housefly makes good use of balancing sticks: a thread with a ball attached to it is implanted under both wings, but if that thread is removed, the creature loses its bearings and starts flying around at random, no longer able to tell top from bottom or left from right—its organ of balance has been destroyed. Man and other mammals are equipped not with balancing sticks but with kinds of tiny stones positioned on hinges in the canals in the inner ear. These canals contain a sticky fluid, which exerts pressure on the stones when the body moves. In people with sensitive organs of balance the stones pop up too violently in response to sudden abrupt movements (shaky elevators, bumpy roads, air pockets during jet flight, swells on a ship). Sometimes sensitivity to balance is so great that even walking ceases to be a pleasurable activity. In that case it is better to get on a bike, since cycling is a more even movement with fewer abrupt changes.

Now for taste. Cows have an extremely thick, undiscriminating tongue. Nevertheless, the cow's taste buds are not indifferent to the quality of the meal: by producing rancid substances, the buttercup is able to save its skin. On the other hand, cats, which are renowned for their fastidiousness, have taste buds that seem to be able to discern even the taste of water.

In short, despite quite far-reaching similarities in form and function, from animal to animal there is great variation in the sensitivity and range of their senses. Henceforward we shall include such facts in the discussion, even though it is difficult to transport ourselves into the world of smell of other animals. Here, a problem arises which has already been mentioned. For example, the range of the wavelengths at which the compound eye of a honeybee can see is between 300 and 650 nanometers, which means that the bee perceives ultraviolet rays but is insensitive to red. The range of the human eye is between 400 and 750 nanometers (violet to red). Young people can hear notes between 20 Hz and 18,000 Hz or more (the "whistle" of the television). While bats are sensitive to sounds ranging from 2,000 to no less than 250,000 Hz, a bat cannot generally hear the human voice (in a conversation the frequencies are mainly around the 1,000 Hz mark).

Also, because smells cannot be grouped under a single common denominator, this kind of comparison cannot be applied without qualification to the organ of smell. It is, however, possible to indicate threshold values which give some indication of the sensitivity to certain substances. For example, in man the threshold value (or detection threshold) for thiol (tetrahydrothiophene, a substance added to natural gas as a warning signal) is 0.4 billion molecules per centiliter. In dogs the value is 0.2 million, giving a difference of a factor of 2,000, so that dogs smell that odor much better.[17] This difference is quite a manageable one. In the case of butyric acid, the ratio is 100 billion units for man as opposed to 9,000 for dogs, giving a difference of a factor of more than 10,000,000. There are very extreme ratios in the case of acetic acid: in man the threshold is around 50,000 billion molecules per centiliter, while the dog requires only 200,000 molecules. On average a dog's sense of smell is several hundred times more sensitive than that of a man. A counterexample is that a human can smell butyl alcohol better than a rat, an animal with a very good sense of smell. Since there are an estimated 400,000 odors that can be distinguished, it is impossible and, moreover, absurd to sum up the threshold values for all those substances.[18] Over the years attempts have been made to introduce some structure by arranging odors into classes, analogous to the way in which light is divided into colors. In Chapter 3 we shall discuss a number of those classifications. In the first instance we shall make do with a tripartite division into types of olfactory organ, partly based on anatomical facts.

Good Smellers, Poor Smellers and Non-smellers

The size of the olfactory organ means nothing: whales have enormous ones, but can smell virtually nothing with them, in contrast to mice, which have the smallest olfactory organs of any mammal yet have an acute sense of smell. In certain types of whale the olfactory organ is of little importance and is (hence?) only moderately developed. Such an animal has little to fear from other species, and for making social contacts it mainly uses its imposing "voice."

Most mammals (rodents, herbivores, many predators) but also fish (eels), amphibians (newts), reptiles (such as snakes) and a few species of birds (pigeons) have a well-developed capacity for smell. For that reason these species are called *macrosmates* (good or great smellers). In relative terms they have an extensive olfactory organ, the epithelium (i.e., the top layer of cells in which the sensory cells are located), which covers a large part of the nasal cavity. The function of a well-developed sense of smell is obvious: a prey is better able to escape the predator; on the other hand the predator can track down its prey more effectively with the aid of a good nose, so the sword cuts both ways. Many mammal macrosmates also have the famous wet nose, which it uses to determine the direction of the wind and to some extent locate odors present in the air.

Insects, too, can generally smell very well; they usually do so with their antennae. These contain numerous pores, where the nerve endings from the sensory cells are located. Insects probably determine the direction of the source of the smell (partly) by moving their antennae. The champion in this area is undoubtedly the male of the silkworm moth (*Bombyx*), which is able to find a sexually available female miles away through the scent bombykol, which she secretes. A concentration of one molecule to one thousand billion units of air would be sufficient to trigger searching behavior in the male. That principle applies to many other animals, such as the pike: this fish hunts with the aid of its eyes and seeks out a mate with the aid of smell.

With *microsmates* (poor or small smellers) the sense of smell is less important. In these animals the nose is proportionately smaller than in macrosmates, the smell epithelium covers only a small section of the nasal cavity, and the number of sensory cells is relatively small. Moreover, the nose is either not at all or scarcely wet, so the animal finds it more difficult to determine the direction of the source of a smell. It will come as no surprise that most birds belong in the category of microsmates. In a bird's life smell is of little significance. The highest concentration of all kinds of smells is found just above ground level, and smells disperse quickly in the open air. In addition, these smells move mainly in a horizontal plane and cling to objects (think of the way such animals as cats mark territory as their own). Sound, in comparison, moves easily through the air, precisely at and from a great height, because of the lack of obstacles up there.

The consequence of this is clear: a blackbird keeps its rivals away more effectively by singing its song high up in a tree than, for example, by marking branches with a smell (nocturnal birds may rely more on hearing and possibly also on smell). One exception to this is the pigeon, one of the few efficient smellers among birds, a creature that may also use odors to get its bearings. Some researchers suspect that pigeons make a kind of *olfactory map* of their surroundings, although there are no solid experimental data to support this hypothesis.[19] Pigeons can still find their way (although slightly less well) if their sense of smell is anesthetized, a fact that appears virtually to demolish attempts to explain their mysterious behavior on the basis of their sense of smell.[20]

Finally, animals without a functioning olfactory organ are called *anosmates* (non-smellers). They live in an odorless world. Usually their olfactory organ is only rudimentary, as with the toothed whale.

Where should we place man along this continuum? The question is difficult to answer. Generally we are regarded as microsmates, but it does not follow from this that our sense of smell is poor. There is something entirely different at issue: we are not *conscious* of many olfactory stimuli. It has already been said: this is because the olfactory nerve has many connections with the ancient limbic system that regulates our feelings and emotions to an important extent, together with the right-hand side of the brain.[21] The limbic system has only limited or indirect connections with language centers, particularly in the newest part of the left cortex. This explains, for example, why so many people find it so difficult to put feelings and emotions into words, and why people are quite often influenced in their behavior by smells without being consciously aware of them.[22]

Nevertheless, in terms of our evolutionary history the situation is complex and confused. Modern man had many precursors which became extinct, some as "side branches." Some researchers suspect that the Neanderthal, like even older precursors, had a better sense of smell than do we, *Homo sapiens sapiens*,[23] whereas "aquatic man" (that is, a hominoid that is supposed to have gained its sustenance mainly from the sea as a "diving mammal") probably had a less well developed sense of smell.[24] A phenomenon which may be connected with this aquatic man or ape is that our nasal canals are seldom both equally easily passable. Some biologists suspect that aquatic man, like all other mammals that derive their food from the water, possessed a muscle that closed off the nostrils when he took to the water. A remnant of that muscle, they argue, might be responsible for the odd behavior of our nostrils. After all, anthropological literature says that primitive peoples smelled better than we do.

The Importance of the Olfactory Organ

Our environment is made up not only of images and sounds, but of olfactory sensations as well. Many aromatic substances circulate in the air in wild confusion, constantly changing in composition, character and intensity. The observation that our environment is also and even mainly a world of smells does not tally with our wont to sing the praises of eye and ear only. In man these senses are well developed indeed. They have connections with many parts of the brain, and the information they provide makes a direct appeal: what we hear and see often preoccupies us. What we smell, in contrast, leads only to short-lived revulsion or delight, or else the perception scarcely impinges on us. However, we must bear in mind that even sensations we are hardly aware of may affect our functioning or behavior profoundly. No one knows exactly *how* he or she walks, for example, but the ability to walk is crucially important in our behavioral repertoire.

The complex of structures in the brain involved in the sense of smell is called the *rhinencephalon* (the smelling brain). In macrosmates the olfactory system occupies a significant part of (total) brain tissue, and smell has a great deal of direct or indirect influence on behavior. So the structure of the smelling brain in man scarcely differs from that in other mammals; it is just that in our case the size of the olfactory system in relation to the total brain mass is comparatively small. To put it another way: the smelling brain is old in evolutionary terms, it has proved important or valuable, and nature has copied or constructed it in our brains on the basis of the animal world. However much variation there may be from mammal to mammal, in the field of smells mammals can be said to speak roughly the same language.

One last point. It is a well-known (if not entirely uncontroversial) fact that evolution more or less repeats itself on a small scale in the embryological development of the individual (Haeckel's law): for example, early stages of a human embryo look strikingly like phases observed in the development of lower animals. This "recapitulation" also applies to the formation of sensory cells and their links with the brain. Not only is the sense of smell old, but it is also laid down early in the brain's development. The olfactory epithelium emerges at a very early fetal stage, after which rapid connections are made with the brain tissue. The other sensory systems emerge only later. In the behavior of the newborn infant the originally prominent role of the olfactory system is gradually taken over more and more by the functions of the other senses and the many other functions of the cerebrum, such as thinking and the use of language.

There are reasons to assume that a child's first sensation is in the sphere of smell. We begin our life, as it were, not by seeing the light of day, but by smelling a kind of "life smell" diffused in the fluid of the womb. There are various pointers in this direction. It is known that rats perceive the smell of their mother in the womb; that turns out to be a precondition for their being able to recognize their mother after birth and to develop full suckling behavior. Moreover, it is known that the imprinting of the smell of the amniotic fluid in rats is also important in their learning to identify their relations.[25] The same principle applies to other species. By suckling their mother's nipples baby mice absorb her body odor; young mice cannot find nipples that have been washed. Young death's-head monkeys have a clear preference for their mother, but that preference disappears if the mother monkey's smell is washed away. Conversely, washed lambs are often not accepted by the ewe and baby rabbits smeared with the scent of a strange female run the risk of being attacked by their mother.[26] In the animal kingdom, then, the bond between parent and offspring is to a large extent made by smell.

Here one could make a (cautious) comparison with the spectacular migration of salmon. Probably the smell of the spawning grounds is perceived and imprinted by the salmon at the embryonic stage, and this is how it can find its way back to the area.[27]

Chapter 2

The Olfactory Organ

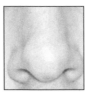

The nose is separated into two cavities by a partition (*septum*); both cavities are divided up into a number of chambers by three nasal *conchae*. This is depicted in Figure 1.[28] Because of the complex structure of the opening, turbulent currents of air are created in the nose, which is one of the reasons why determining the exact dosage of a fragrance to be administered meets with difficulties.[29] One might think that for proper administering and measurement it would be desirable for there to be a constant stream of air across the sensory cells of the olfactory epithelium. This is wrong: the olfactory organ operates efficiently only when there is a certain level of *varied* stimulus; this is probably why the turbulence exists. In the case of smell that variation is provided in two ways: there is turbulence in the nostrils and we have a tendency to sniff when we (think we) smell something. The same principle applies to sight. When the spontaneous tiny eye movements that provide a varied stimulus to the retina are blocked (for example, with the aid of so-called stabilized images), the person is virtually blind.[30]

Moreover, the olfactory organ is stimulated by two, and in the-

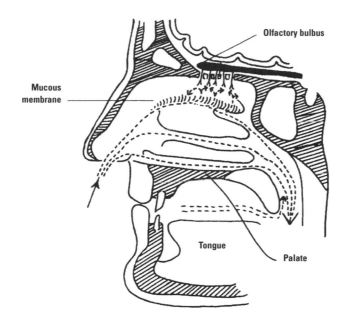

**Figure 1. Cross section of part of the head. The olfactory
organ is located at the top of the nasal cavity. The arrows
indicate the direction of the current of air in nasal breathing.
During eating, air also passes from the mouth to
the olfactory organ.**

ory even three, routes: the nasal cavity is connected with the outside air through the nostrils and with the "inner air" via the throat
(the nasopharynx). In this way smells also penetrate the olfactory
organ via the mouth, during meals, for example. It is also possible
to smell (and taste) substances via injections; tiny amounts of these
find their way into the organ of olfaction via the bloodstream.

Smell and Taste

Generally, the sense of smell turns out to have a great deal of
influence on the perception and appreciation of tastes. The sense
of taste is reinforced and influenced by smell, because during eating air is forced upward from the mouth through chewing movements. People who eat with blocked noses taste only a few

flavors—namely, sweet, sour, salty and bitter. Smell is largely responsible for a full perception of taste. For example, research has shown that coffee loses a lot of its flavor and indeed is no longer recognizable as coffee if the nose is blocked.[31] In such cases a loss of recognizability, sometimes to as low as 10 percent of optimum value (Figure 2), also occurs with other foods, beverages and spices, such as wine, sugared water, cherries, apricot, pineapple, chocolate, syrup, cinnamon and garlic.[32] Even with water, recognizability is reduced, though to a limited degree.

It can also be deduced from this why colds adversely affect the taste of food and drink. The swelling of the mucous layer of the nasal epithelium leads to the obstruction of the passage of air across the organ of olfaction, so that smells are less able to penetrate to the sensory cells effectively. In short, the experience of taste is to a significant degree determined by smells; a good supply of air to the organ of olfaction is essential in order to be able to enjoy a meal. Another remarkable fact can be mentioned in this connection. Food odors that reach the organ of olfaction via the oral cavity are somewhat different in quality than those inhaled directly. Think, for example, of the smell of a boiled egg compared with the combination of the smell and taste of the egg as we eat it. It is possible that the *direction* of the current of air is important to the way in which the sense of smell functions—namely, directly or via the mouth. Another possibility is that the two senses interact in a complex way.[33] It is also clear that the concentration of odor molecules in the air is different (and probably higher, because we inhale the smell) than the smells which reach the organ of olfaction via the nasopharynx; the composition of the latter may be different as a consequence of chewing and the action of saliva, so that other molecules emerge and pass through the nasopharynx. (See Chapter 3 for the consequences of a change in concentration for the experience of smell.)

Apart from etiquette, there is a good reason not to talk with one's mouth full: it means a loss of precious smells making their way to the organ of olfaction. Smoking during a meal also has an adverse effect on the experience of taste. This is because certain substances in tobacco smoke stimulate the trigeminal nerve (of

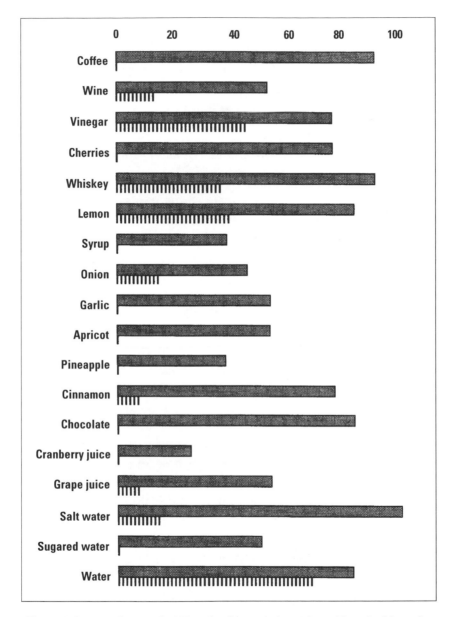

Figure 2. Degree of recognizability of substances in tasting with and without the involvement of the olfactory organ. If access to the olfactory organ is blocked (lower bar on histogram), recognizability is greatly reduced in virtually all substances.

which more below), as a result of which the sense of smell is somewhat inhibited. On the other hand, there are also fragrances in tobacco smoke that for some people can positively affect the overall "taste picture" of a meal. The fact that a cigarette tastes particularly good *after* a meal is easy to explain: because smell and taste have largely lost their sensitivity to the food (through adaptation), a new stimulus makes maximum impact.

The Nasal Cavity and the Olfactory Organ

The nasal cavity is kept moist by a large number of glands. The lateral nasal gland or steno gland is the largest of these; this secretes via a duct to a point near the tip of the nose.[34] Consequently, when we pick our nose this is the point where there is the most matter to be removed. Glandular secretion keeps the nose moist. Not only is this better for breathing (trapping dust particles) but in moist air you also smell more efficiently, because more of an odor can be absorbed. Apart from keeping the air moist, it is suspected that mucus has an additional function: it's possible that fragrances are dissolved in mucus and subsequently carried in the direction of the organ of olfaction. In that way the concentration of the smell can at the same time be increased, since a watery solution can contain many more smell molecules than air. The actual organ of smell is at the top of the nose, a little below eye height, at about the same depth as the palate and approximately three inches from the nostril of an average nose.[35]

Our knowledge of the anatomy, physiology and operation of the organ of olfaction is fairly limited. The main reason for this is that it is difficult to obtain access to it with surgical instruments. It is possible to scrape cells from the epithelium with a kind of crochet needle, but because of the location of the epithelium just below the perforated ethmoid bone in the floor of the cranium, this procedure is quite risky and remains the preserve of skilled surgeons. In experiments with animals in this field, frogs and rats are most commonly used. Their noses are relatively easy to reach with the scalpel. Frogs are used for cruder work such as amputations, rats for behavioral experiments.[36]

In determining the exact anatomy of the organ of olfaction, then, researchers have based their conclusions principally on examination of cadavers or on animal experiments. The statistical data on the human olfactory organ—the size of the epithelium, the thickness of the mucous layer, the number of nerve cells and suchlike—have been shown to be unreliable and require regular adjustment. However, it is certain that the organ of olfaction is small: its surface area covers only approximately one square centimeter per nostril (the retinas in the eye are considerably larger).[37] In young people the surface area may be larger; with the passage of the years the size of the organ of olfaction decreases.

The nasal epithelium contains approximately 30,000 neurons per square millimeter, quite regularly distributed at intervals of between 3 and 5 micrometers. Given the surface area per nostril, the epithelium contains an estimated 3 to 5 million sensory cells, so that left and right together contain between 6 and 10 million. That seems a reasonable number, but if we compare our noses with those of the macrosmates, the picture changes dramatically: a dog's nose, depending on the breed, contains some 150 million (fox terrier) to 220 million cells (sheep dog), while rabbits have 50 million.[38] (The retinas of our eyes contain as a rule more than 200 million light-sensitive rods and cones.) This is why dogs are used for tracking and to sniff out gas leaks underground.

The organ of olfaction as a whole is constructed of a mucous layer, the nasal epithelium (the actual organ of smell) and a supporting layer. Not very much is known about the composition of the mucus. At any rate, this layer is completely unrelated to white or green nasal mucus, which derives from the nasal glands and the respiratory epithelium. The mucous layer of the organ of smell is yellowy brown in color because of the presence of a pigment; its function is not known. Both the thickness and the viscosity of the layer are fairly variable. These variations affect the degree to which fragrances are absorbed from the air inhaled. Many more molecules can be dissolved in water than in air, which even applies to hydrophobic substances: the solubility coefficient in water is greater than that in air by a factor of between 10 and 1,000.[39] The composition and hence the odor-dissolving capacity of the

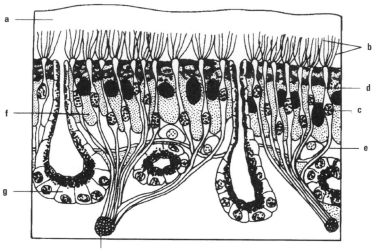

Figure 3. Schematic structure of the olfactory organ. Located in the mucous layer (a) are the olfactory cilia (b) of the sensory cells. These cells consist of a cellular body (c), a dendrite (d) and a neurite or axon (e). They are wedged in between support cells (f). The mucous layer is maintained by Bowman's glands (g).

mucous layer is influenced by a large number of factors. A simple cold blocks the flow of air across the olfactory organ because of the swelling of the mucous layer; the layer itself becomes thicker and its viscosity changes, with the result that this kind of transportation of molecules to the olfactory organ is largely stopped. It is also conceivable that the smell-binding capacity of the mucus is effected. Finally, hormones can be shown to affect the thickness of the layer; this might be one of the explanations for the fact that women exhibit a markedly varying sensitivity to fragrances in the course of the menstrual cycle.[40]

The epithelium of the organ of olfaction consists of three kinds of cells: sensory cells, support cells and basal cells (see Figure 3).[41] The sensory cells are *naked neurons*, which means that they are in direct contact with the outside world (the nasal cavity), although embedded in mucus. Direct exposure to the outside air means that a sensory cell has a limited lifetime. After four to eight weeks it is worn out and replaced by a new cell. This arrangement creates another problem: certain pathogenic or poisonous substances, as well as viruses, can find their way into the brain via the sensory cells, often with harmful effects. This, again, was a subject of much debate in earlier times.[42]

The oblong olfactory sensory cell is a *bipolar neuron*, or a cell with two branching processes, a dendrite and a neurite. (By comparison, the unipolar rods and cones in the retina have no dendrites or branching processes.) A dendrite moves in the direction of the source (i.e., the stimulus, the cause); a neurite passes the information on and hence forms a connection between the source and the eventual processing of the information in the brain. The dendrites of the neuron meet in a node—the axon node—which carries between ten and thirty olfactory hairs implanted in a crisscross pattern. Olfactory hairs can be compared to a kind of hairlike cilium, containing tiny tubes (*microtubili*), which are also found in the rods and cones in the retina. The actual receptors are found in these olfactory hairs. This was established, for example, in an experiment in which the nasal epithelium of a frog was treated with Triton X-100), a special substance that extracts the olfactory hairs while leaving the rest of the epithelium intact.[43] As a result, the electrical activity of the sensory organ, as represented in an electro-olfactogram (EOG), is completely eliminated, so that the presence of olfactory hairs is a necessary precondition for the ability to smell.

The pear-shaped brush cells occur in a proportion of one to between ten and twenty sensory cells. The brush cells stand out because of the large number of *microvilli*, microscopic protuberances (which explains their name). The function of these cells is not known; perhaps, because of their position in the olfactory organ, they are involved in the removal of mucus and the breakdown of dead sensory cells (similar brush cells also occur in the respiratory epithelium). In rats and other rodents brush cells are found in large numbers in another organ in the nasal cavity, the *vomeronasal organ* (discussed below).

The bottle-shaped support cells make up the greater part of the mass of the nasal epithelium, which means that the majority of the cells in the organ of olfaction make no contribution to smell in the strict sense. The support cells form a matrix in which the neurons are embedded at regular intervals, like corn in a field. Like the brush cells, the support cells also carry large numbers of microvilli. In addition, these cells also carry a certain kind of mucus, and probably they are also involved in the removal of harmful substances from the support layer. These cells probably also play a part in the manufacture and "recycling" of the so-called odorant-binding proteins.

The small basal cells on the underside of the epithelium are able to replace degenerated sensory cells. Though the taste buds in the papillae on the tongue can also do this, they are not neurons. In the olfactory organ we are dealing with true *neurogenesis*—that is, the ability to create new nerve tissue to replace old. This is not a superfluous luxury: we have already observed that an olfactory sensory cell is in the firing line. The cell is in direct contact with inhaled substances that are alien to the body and sometimes harmful, which means that it has a short life. The process of replacement operates roughly as follows (Figure 4).[44]

At a certain moment the basal cell is stimulated to divide. The "daughter nuclei" move slowly in the direction of the mucous layer, and a dendrite and a neurite are formed. When the neurite is able to establish contact with the rhinencephalon via other nerves, the dendrite produces olfactory hairs and the new sensory cell becomes operational. How the contact between the cell and the brain is established is a mystery that neurobiology has not yet been able to solve.[45] It may be a process of trial and error, since only sensory cells able to make the right connections survive; the others die off. Thanks to this exceptional regenerative ability a damaged organ of olfaction can repair itself, even if this involves making connections with the associated portions of the brain: the basal cells make new neurons, and these form connections with other cells. Basal cells have even been grown successfully in a culture and allowed to develop into olfactory sensory cells.

Even if an essential component of the rhinencephalon, the *bulbus olfactorius*, is removed, the sensory cells are able to recover after a period of decline, provided the nerve endings of the nasal

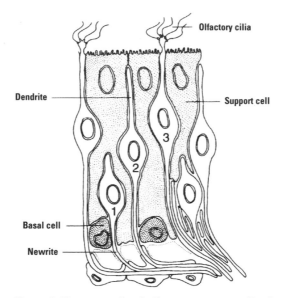

Figure 4. Neurogenesis of olfactory sensory cells. A basal cell divides, creating new neurons (stage 1). When the cells link up with the olfactory nerve, they move in the direction of the mucous layer and also form a dendrite (stage 2). A sensory cell with olfactory cilia gradually emerges (stage 3).

epithelium are not cut off. Sometimes the fibers of the sensory cells reestablish contact with the brain, which eventually leads to some recovery of smell. As far as is known, only olfactory sensory cells are capable of neurogenesis. The flexibility of the olfactory system is indeed so great that damage to a part of the rhinencephalon in animals like mice and rats leads to a repair of the brain, which is not the case in parts of the brain concerned with the other senses.[46] Even transplantations of the olfactory epithelium to another area in the brain (again in the case of damage), for example, are possible. The implanted tissue continues growing and the cells acquire branching processes, which make contact with the surrounding brain tissue, so that certain functions can be restored.[47] In other words, the organ of olfaction is so multifunctional that olfactory sensory cells can take over tasks in damaged portions of the brain, which means that the cells can also be useful in other places. These are remarkable findings, in view of the fact that until recently the assumption was that lost brain and sensory cells are not replaced.

From an evolutionary perspective, however, these facts can be understood. The lower an animal's position on the phylogenetic ladder, the more damage it can withstand: for example, a worm that is cut in half develops into two distinct individuals. Perhaps the capacity for self-repair in the organ of olfaction and the rhinencephalon is due to the fact that this sense and the associated parts of the brain are so old in evolutionary terms.

However, there is also a downside to the regenerative capacity of the organ of olfaction. Dangerous substances that are absorbed by the olfactory hairs and that—usually as a result of continuing stimulation—are not adequately removed remain in the olfactory epithelium. As a result of the rapid process of division of the base cells, these substances can make their way quite quickly to the brain and damage the nerve tissue. Apparently there is a core of truth in the dangers, mentioned in Chapter 1, which were supposed to be associated with inhaling certain unpleasant smells, especially if the concentration is quite high and one is confronted with the smell on a daily basis (see Chapters 4 and 8).

Beneath the sensory epithelium there is another supporting layer, the *lamina propria*, that connects the organ of olfaction to the ethmoid bone. Here are located *Bowman's glands*; the secretion duct of these glands runs through the epithelium. The function of these glands is not clear; perhaps like the support cells they play a part in the production of odorant-binding proteins, which will be discussed below. There are also blood vessels in the lamina propria, and the axons of the sensory cells are joined here into nodes which combine to form the olfactory nerve or first brain nerve.

The Operation of a Sensory Cell

In the literature on the psychology of perception a distinction is made between external events, processes which affect a sense (*perireceptor events*), and processes which take place in the sensory cell itself (*receptor events*).[48]

Many factors play roles in the absorption of smells by the mucous layer in the olfactory epithelium. First, the solubility of the odor is important: hydrophobic substances, fatty substances like musk, for example, dissolve easily in the mucous layer. Second, the molecular weight of the odors is important: large molecules have greater difficulty moving through the current of air and they are absorbed less quickly into the mucous layer. Third, the absorption of odors depends partly on the viscosity of the mucus. Another factor is the thickness of the mucous layer. The larger this layer, the greater the distance between the receptors and the source of the odor, and the speed of reaction of the organ of olfaction decreases accordingly. On the other hand, a thicker layer of mucus means a larger number of olfactory hairs, as a result of which the number of points of attachment for the substances increases.

Strictly speaking, the organ of olfaction has to deal with the same kind of problem as the body's immune system. How can a distinction be made between alien and non-alien substances, between odors which indicate something useful and those which are harmful? This is not easy to decide. As has been noted, fatty, heavy molecules encounter many problems in transportation in the direction of the sensory cell, although they often contain important information—for example, on body odors. Thus it is in the interests of the organism to offer such molecules a helping hand.

This line of thinking has resulted in recent years in a meticulous search for constituents in the mucus and the epithelium whose operation is similar to that of the immune system. For example, some years ago it was discovered that the mucous layer and the cell membrane of the olfactory hairs contain a protein which can bind odorants to it. Such a protein has up to now been found only in the organ of olfaction; hence the name *odorant-binding protein* or OBP (sometimes also OMP, *olfactory marker protein*, or OR, *olfactory receptor*). An odorant-binding protein which has since been identified consists of 172 amino acids and has a molecular weight of over 18,000. In view of the fact that in humans there is often a specific anosmia or inability to smell which occurs only with regard to certain substances, it is assumed by various researchers that there will be more such proteins operating in the mucus and in the cell membrane. Up until now, however, no other odorant-binding proteins have been found; moreover, it has proved difficult to identify potential chemical candidates as specific odorant-binding substances.[49]

As things look at present, an odorant-binding protein has two functions. In the first place, it facilitates the dissolving of odorants in the mucous layer. It also ensures that there is no oversaturation: the protein also operates as a kind of safety system. The moderate production of this protein by glands in the nose, a process which precedes their absorption into the mucous layer, may be compatible with this assumption. It is also conceivable that the protein is used to remove odorants after they have done their work. The production of odorant-binding protein by the support cells, and by the glands present in the supporting layer of the organ of olfaction, might point in this direction. In addition, the protein appears to be important in stimulating electrical activity, which goes hand in hand with the operation of the neurons. Strictly speaking, this process forms part of the receptor events, which will now be discussed in greater detail.

Precisely how an odorant stimulates a sensory cell is still not clear. With the discovery of the odorant-binding protein, it was thought that a specific receptive molecule had been found (located in the membrane of the olfactory hairs) which binds odorants to it. This "receptor protein hypothesis" assumes that the connections made by the odorants with the odorant-binding protein affect the enzymatic properties of this protein (that is, properties which stimulate chemical reactions; Figure 5).

The odorant-binding protein activated by the odorant binds a G protein, which in turn aids the catalytic effect of the enzyme adenyl cyclase (AC). This enzyme converts ATP (adenosine triphosphate, a high-energy molecular compound found in many cells) into cyclical AMP (adenosine monophosphate), or cAMP, which operates as a second information carrier and converts other proteins in turn. These include proteins in the ion ducts in the

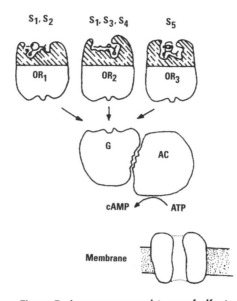

S_1, S_2 S_1, S_3, S_4 S_5

OR$_1$ OR$_2$ OR$_3$

G   AC

cAMP   ATP

Membrane

Figure 5. there are several types of olfactory
sensory cells (S) in which it is suspected
various odorant-binding proteins (here
identified as OR) are active. When such a
protein binds an odorant molecule, it is
activated. It attaches to a G protein,
eventually converting ATP into cAMP. This
substance opens the ion ducts in the
membrane, activating the nerve and creating
the olfactory sensation.

membrane, which are opened by the reaction with cAMP. As a result of this, positively charged atoms (sodium and potassium) are admitted to the cell. If that happens in various places, the olfactory hair membrane becomes depolarized. The cAMP ensures that the operation of the odorant-binding protein is inhibited, which means that there is feedback in the system. To summarize a complicated process: an odorant activates the protein; subsequently there is a chain reaction, which leads to an electrical discharge by the olfactory hair membrane; eventually the activation is terminated by the odorant-binding protein.

Unfortunately, a number of phenomena conflict with the receptor protein hypothesis.[50] Some odorants precisely *lower* the electrical activity in the neurons; in that case even fewer discharges occur than in a resting state (every sensory cell also displays spontaneous electrical activity when resting). In addition the hypothesis, while it presents a plausible picture of how an odorant opens ion ducts, does not suggest how it closes them. The effect of combinations of smells is also difficult to explain in this way. The constituents of a mixture may reinforce one another's operation; in that case, the number of discharges must be greater than the sum of discharges when the odorants are presented separately. This fact does not tally with the idea of a proportional binding by the receptor proteins: in the latter case, the number of discharges can never exceed the sum of the separate effects.

Another problem is how one is to explain the extreme *variation* in the sensitivity of the olfactory organ. During its four-day fertility cycle, the maximum sensitivity to butyric acid in female mice is a million times greater than minimum sensitivity, although the quantity of receptor protein(s) remains virtually constant. Hence there are probably other mechanisms involved besides odorant-binding proteins. To mention only one example: a smell can cause the composition of the mucous layer to change, which may influence the electrical activity of the neurons. In addition, the blood vessels in the supporting layers sometimes react to certain odors; that can also have (indirect) consequences for the pattern of discharge of the nerve fibers. Finally, it is possible that the metabolism of the cells in the epithelium is affected by certain odorants. However, the operation of all those processes is far from clear.

One of the few indications that other factors may be involved besides the operation of odorant-binding proteins is the following. The substance adenyl cyclase (AC), which normally catalyzes the conversion of ATP into cAMP, turns out to be particularly active in the olfactory hairs—namely, fifteen times more active than in membranes belonging to brain cells. The AC in the olfactory hairs has a specific effect; it doesn't operate on ATP, but on GTP (guanine triphosphate), a substance also found in other sensory systems. The AC converts GTP into cAMP, which then opens the ion ducts and so indirectly drains the membrane. When odorants are applied to the olfactory hairs of a frog, the activity of the AC is shown to increase at higher concentrations of the odorant (provided GTP is available), but the same experiment has no effect when applied to the membrane of brain cells. In short, the activity of the AC in the olfactory-hair membranes depends on the odorants absorbed, and the receptor proteins do not have a monopoly on the conversion of odor molecules into electrical signals. Ultimately, all the membrane discharges are integrated; every sensory cell has a number of olfactory hairs, whose signals converge at the axon node. The more ion ducts are opened onto these olfactory hairs and hence the more discharges that take place, the more electrical impulses will be given out by the sensory cell ("firing"). In this way, the signal is transmitted to the next connection via the nerve fibers. This is found in the brain, in the olfactory bulbus.

The Rhinencephalon

This structure of the brain originates in a tube closed at one end, which in the course of evolution has acquired bulges. The rhinencephalon includes the two bulbi olfactorii (BO); two rods with a bulge; and also the olfactory cortex. The BO were formed at the end of the tube, a process that took place far back in evolutionary history—BO are already found in insects. In sharks the construction can still clearly be seen, but in man the most recent parts of the cortex have, as it were, grown over the remnants of the tube. The bulbus parts occupy on average only one-tenth of 1 percent of the brain volume in man—no more than 1.4 milliliters out of a content of approximately 1.4 liters.

Via perforations in the ethmoid bone in the skull, the sensory cells make contact with the BO, aided by neurites. This is where the first processing of the signals from the sensory cells takes place, a process that subsequently occurs in the olfactory cortex. In the latter area, the signals are analyzed and linked with other information. In the neocortex the sense of smell mainly affects the general activity of the right brain; the implications of this will be discussed below. A further observation that can be made is that not only was the rhinencephalon laid down at an early stage but it is fairly certain that *stimulation* of the organ of olfaction is essential to the development of the corresponding part of the brain.[51]

The finger-shaped BO is built up from six layers (Figure 6),[52] the structure and organization of which show marked similarities to those of the retina.[53] The nerve fibers converge into the glomeruli, switch boxes where the signals are connected. The human BO has approximately 1,000 such areas. Given the number of sensory cells for each olfactory organ (we are working on the assumption of approximately three million), this means that on average for each smell sensation no fewer than three thousand signals have to be processed by a single glomerulus. Because the whole is more or less spatially organized, it is sometimes claimed that smelling involves a kind of "olfactory space" originating in the bulbus, and that this may reflect the position of the sensory cells in the organ of olfaction—a principle that also applies to other senses. It might be possible to demonstrate that there are differences in the reactions of sensory cells to different groups of odorants, depending on the *place* where the substances stimulate the olfactory organ, although there is no question of an exact one-to-one correspondence between the position of the sensory cell and the position of entry of the signal in the BO.[54] The indications for the existence of an olfactory space are few, since it is technically very difficult to trace the signals of separate groups of sensory cells in the bulbus.[55]

The olfactory cortex (OC) consists of a number of sections, of which the olfactory nucleus, located toward the front, is the most important. Because of its less thick and less complex structure, the OC can easily be distinguished from the surrounding structures in the (neo)cortex. The OC also has a layered structure, although this is less pronounced with the BO. The information from the BO (which, topographically, is reasonably well ordered) is spread across the OC in a varied mosaic, which seems to rule out the link between the spatial organization in the olfactory epithelium and

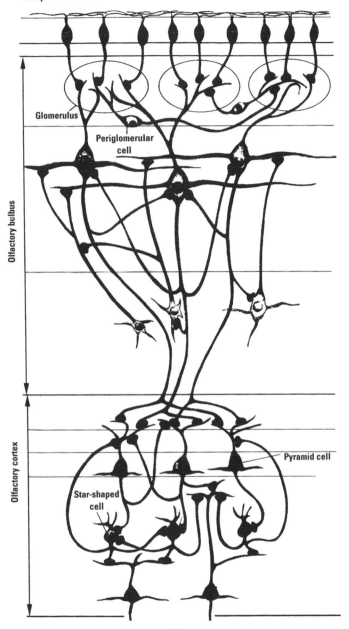

Receptors in the nose

Glomerulus

Periglomerular cell

Olfactory bulbus

Olfactory cortex

Pyramid cell

Star-shaped cell

Figure 6. Schematic structure of the olfactory bulbus and cortex. Integration of the signals takes place in the glomeruli. The periglomerular cells are responsible for inhibiting processes. Next the signals are transmitted via several other types of cells to pyramid cells in the cortex. The star-shaped cells are thought to be responsible for the creation or establishing of associations.

that of the signal codes. It is suspected that not only spatial organization but also a time dimension is involved in the processing
of smells: possibly the OC makes a kind of three-dimensional
(space-time) model of the sensation of smell.[56] Little of the fairly
strict hierarchical organization in the BO is found in the OC.[57]
There is some system or order: the neurons on the surface transfer
information mainly to the neocortex, while the nerve cells, which
are situated more deeply, mainly make connections with the thalamus, the hypothalamus and parts of the limbic system (which is
closely connected with feelings and emotions), such as the *amyg-
dala*. The links between the CO and the neocortex are proportionately few; some consequences of this will be discussed in
Chapter 5.

In the research into information processing in the OC, radio-
active substances are currently being used to trace and map nerve
connections, but little has been learned so far. We do know that
four kinds of switching mechanisms occur in the OC;[58] to simplify,
some switches analyze and decode the smell and other switches
ensure that an actual *sensation* of smell takes place consciously
or unconsciously.

The Trigeminal Nerve

The olfactory organ does not have a monopoly on smelling odors;
there are two competitors. The *trigeminal nerve* (the fifth cranial
nerve) is primarily responsible for "feeling" in the face. In mammals this nerve also reacts to certain chemical substances, including smells.[59] In addition, many mammals have a *vomeronasal
organ*, which is at the front of the nose and is linked by a duct
with the oral cavity. This organ also has a certain capacity for
smell.[60] People who because of damage to or dysfunction of the
olfactory organ can smell scarcely or not at all, can generally perceive the sharp smell of ammonia, for example. The extremities
of the trigeminal nerve are responsible for these kinds of sensations.

As the name indicates, this nerve has three main paths, which enter the face at eye height. The main branches run to the fore-head, the cheeks and the nose—including the nasal cavities as well as the oral cavity and the chin. In the nasal cavities and the mouth the nerve divides into a large number of small branches which register specifically (dental) pain, heat and irritation; the ends of the branches are linked to receptors sensitive to temperature, pressure and touch. Many of the extremities are "free"—that is, not equipped with specific receptors. In high concentrations these branching processes are also stimulated by odorants. This happens especially when confronted with dangerous substances: these lead to irritation or pain. The general function of the trigeminal nerve will be clear: this nerve protects us against harmful external influences. This is why the perception of a substance like ammonia leads to a general repellent reaction.

Olfactory research generally disregards the trigeminal system. This is a mistake: clearly there is an interplay between the olfactory system and the trigeminal nerve.[61] Many substances, like alcohol, turpentine, amylobutyric acid, but also the less pungent carbon dioxide, are perceived by both systems. It is remarkable that the olfactory organ should also and mainly react to *low* concentrations of odorants. After the threshold value has been passed and the trigeminal system is activated we find that the olfactory organ (despite the greatly increased quantity) scarcely notices the odor. In other words, with an increasing strength of stimuli, smelling proper often gives way to a kind of alarm function in the form of pain and/or irritation; in that case, the trigeminal system mutes the signals from the olfactory organ somewhat, possibly because the sense of smell would otherwise be damaged. The fact that the trigeminal system is connected with danger also emerges from the fact that a non-aggressive odor inhibits the activity of the trigeminal system, which fits neatly into the hypothesis. Moreover, for this reason we must be cautious in interpreting the differences in the smelling capacity in men and women, the young and the old, smokers and non-smokers: the interaction between the olfactory and the trigeminal system may be a contributing factor. It is not impossible, for example, that an olfactory organ which functions less well is often associated with heightened sensitivity of the trigeminal system: a cold can intensify the aversion to cigarette smoke even in heavy smokers.

A strange property of the trigeminal nerve is its sensitivity to "addiction," and aversion can even be converted into preference. Examples of this are cocaine, tobacco smoke, pepper, mustard, curry, ginger, horseradish and vinegar, substances that strongly stimulate the trigeminal nerve. The sniffing of solvents (glue) probably belongs here, too. Children and adults confronted for the first time with pepper, for example, show an aversion. After repeated confrontations, however, the aversion frequently changes to a preference. An explanation for this might be that pepper stimulates the digestion and is actually harmless, although the body in the first instance has an adverse reaction.

With cocaine and to a lesser extent tobacco smoke something else is involved: the odors that are not inhaled are often unpleasant, but the inhaled smoke or powder results in a kind of euphoric effect in the central nervous system. The eventual harmful effects are not linked in a sensory or direct way with sniffing or smoking. In the first instance, these substances provoke pleasant sensations, and possible punishment results only after many years. A stimulus which in the first instance produces pleasant effects may be strongly preferred, via a process of "sensation seeking."[62] The neurophysiological origin of these phenomena is unclear. In addition, one cannot say that the change in the appreciation of a smell is a general principle in the animal kingdom: for example, it has not been possible to create a preference for pepper in rats.

The Vomeronasal Organ

The vomeronasal organ (also known as Jacobson's organ) has an important function in rodents, grazing animals and carnivores. This cigar-shaped organ is at the front of the nasal cavity. In dogs and horses there is an aperture between the upper lip and the front teeth which leads to the *nasopalatine duct* (*canalis nasopalatinis*), which connects the vomeronasal organ and the mouth. In mice and other rodents that aperture is directly behind the incisors in the palate, as in cats. In the latter this can be seen easily: hold the cat's mouth open and look behind the small incisors. In the palate there is a hole with a slightly raised lid, as in a bathtub. This is the aperture of the connecting duct.

Cats use this organ to investigate body odors and urine more closely. They raise their top lip and upper jaw, so that the odorants can be absorbed more easily. Urine and other substances that evaporate either very little or not at all are sucked in and then tested for their nature and composition by the vomeronasal organ. There are strong indications that this organ is important in the animal kingdom in perceiving stimuli with a decidedly social or sexual meaning (Chapter 6). In horses the raising of the top lip and jaw is called the *flehmen response*. The vomeronasal organ is also laid down in humans in embryonic development, but a few months later it disappears; the organ is present in rudimentary form. We still have the duct in question behind our front incisors; a nerve connected with feeling in the palate runs through it.

The structure of the sensory epithelium of the vomeronasal organ is somewhat similar to that of the olfactory epithelium. One difference is that the sensory cells have no olfactory hairs, but do have microvilli; they are very similar to the brush cells in the olfactory epithelium. It is assumed that the two organs developed independently for a long time; one indication of this might be that Jacobson's organ is already found in reptiles such as snakes.

It is still not clear exactly how the sensory process works. Apart from connections with the organ of olfaction the vomeronasal organ has its own connections with the rhinencephalon; a number of nerve pathways also lead through perforations in the ethmoid bone to other structures in the brain. In a part of the olfactory bulbus specifically reserved for this organ, the signals are processed and transmitted to the hypothalamus and other areas of importance to (the expression of) emotions, including aggression and sexual behavior. As already noted, the vomeronasal organ is used mainly to obtain a first, rapid and often decisive impression of smells that belong in a social and sexual context. Such smells are imprinted at a relatively early stage in life. If the organ is removed after the imprinting stage, it turns out that the nose can cope by itself thereafter. In rats at least, no striking changes in social behavior appear.[63] However, in mice, if *both* the organ of olfaction and the vomeronasal organ are removed, the animals no longer mate, and in females the womb also degenerates.[64]

Chapter 3

The Nature of Smell

How are odorants and sensations of smell linked? That question must be divided into two parts. The quantitative link between one and the other describes the degree to which the intensity of a smell impression increases as the intensity of the stimulus is increased. In theory this relation may take many forms: linear, logarithmic, exponential, random and the like.

Qualitative relationships, however, concern the question of how a smell impression relates to the chemical properties of a substance, whether or not it is included in a mixture. To make this clearer: the color red corresponds to light with a wavelength of approximately 700 millimicrons, and a bleep is based on vibrations of the air with a frequency of roughly 10,000 per second. So it is a matter, then, of what physical or chemical factors are responsible for the properties of a smell sensation. With smell, one determining factor in smell sensation may be the shape of the molecule.

Psychophysics

Such questions have been and continue to be posed for every sense: this brings us into the area of psychophysics. This subsection of perceptual psychology maps connections between all kinds of stimuli and the corresponding sensations. Research up to now has been focused mainly on the eye and the ear, since in these senses both the stimulus and the reaction are relatively easy to measure (moreover, these senses were traditionally highly regarded).

The field of the psychophysics of smell was pioneered by the celebrated Dutch scientist Zwaardemaker at the end of the previous century. Another important Dutch researcher, Stuiver, built the first advanced olfactometer. This is an instrument in which a constant and pure current of air is produced, enabling the researcher to administer a precisely regulated concentration of an odorant.[65]

An olfactometer is an important aid in smell research. The apparatus consists of a complex system of tubes, hoses and pressure vessels, which make it possible to expose each nostril to a precise dosage of an odor. The construction of an olfactometer is complicated partly by the fact that the apparatus must be and remain odorless inside.[66]

One of the first steps to be taken, however, was a different one—namely, the classification of smells. In 1803 the department of "research into sensory perceptions and ideas" was set up in the Institute de France.[67] It was believed that the creation of a language to describe smell sensations would be a means of separating smell from associations with the animal component in human beings. The venture produced unsatisfactory results. Classifying smells turns out to be a problem: smells cannot be lumped together on the basis of common physical or chemical properties, in contrast to visual and auditory stimuli, which are expressed in wavelength or number of vibrations per second (nanometers or millimicrons, Hertz) and intensity (lux, decibel).

Other topics which we will discuss are the adaptation or conditioning to smells and the related variation in sensitivity of the sense of smell, as well as habituation to smells, a kind of process of conditioning or boredom. We also will pay attention to the perception of mixtures of smells, stench and "directional smelling."

Classifying Smells

If one wants to put smells into classes, one can base one's system either on smell impressions or on the chemical properties, molecular structure or shape of the substances. Although in principle the two starting points need not be contradictory, in practice they often lead to divergent results. The hope is that eventually the different classifications can be reconciled, but we are still a long way from that at present.

Plants and animals have a double designation: a generic and a species name. This binary nomenclature derives from the Swede Linnaeus (1707–78), who devised a taxonomic system for plants that is still used today. It struck Linnaeus that plants could also be distinguished on the basis of their scents. He divided scent impressions into seven classes, arranged in descending order of pleasant ("hedonic") quality:[68]

- Aromatic
- Scented or perfumed
- Ambrosia or musk-like
- Sharp or garlic-like
- Stinking or goat-like, sweaty
- Repulsive
- Disgusting

Linnaeus also maintained that certain plant smells are reminiscent of bodily smells. That was supposed to apply particularly to the smell of the genital organs and their secretions. According to him, the hawthorn and various kinds of roses smell like the female pubes. Vaginal secretions, partly depending on the phase in the menstrual cycle, are sometimes less sweet-smelling. Linnaeus associated this smell with that of the stinking goosefoot, which he accordingly called *Chenopodium vulvaria* (some people claim this plant also smells like rotting herring).[69] In addition, the flowers of the elderberry, the lime tree and the chestnut all have a sweet, rather sickly smell, which according to Linnaeus is reminiscent of the smell of sperm; according to him, in those days a preferred spot for proposals of marriage was under chestnut trees. In his opinion, the pollen grains of many types of grass spread a similar kind of smell.

This kind of association is also found in a story by the Marquis de Sade.[70] A girl who has been brought up carefully and in a sheltered home is discussing the smell of chestnut flowers with her mother. The smell is very familiar to her, but she can't place it properly, much to the dismay of a young priest who is visiting, and with whom she had an affair.

Zwaardemaker further refined and expanded Linnaeus's categories. He distinguished nine classes; each class in turn is further subdivided.[71] We shall list only the main classes here, with a few examples:

- Ethereal: acetone, chloroform, ether
- Aromatic: camphor, lavender, menthol, bay, lemon
- Balsamic: vanilla, lily, jasmine and other fresh flower smells
- Amber-like: musk, pheromones such as androstenol and copuline (Chapter 6)
- Alliaceous (from *allium*, garlic): thiol compounds, amines (compounds containing ammonia), rotten eggs, bromide
- Empyreumatic (from *empyreus*, fiery): coffee, toasted bread, tobacco smoke, tar, naphtha, gasoline
- Hircine (from *hircus*, goat): cheese, sweat, urine, particularly cat urine
- Repulsive or suffocating: species in the nightshade family, such as belladonna, bittersweet, crab apple, potato, tomato, pepper, tobacco (the leaves and berries of these plants are often poisonous); coriander, certain orchids, bugs (possessing stink glands), narcotic substances
- Disgusting: rotting flesh and cadaverous odors, indole (an organic compound found, for example, in coal tar), skatole

(produced in the bacterial breakdown of proteins that is also found in feces), predatory flowers (of the genus *Stapelia*, belonging to the silk plant family; these attract flies for pollination with a kind of carrion smell.

This classification is still in use. One continuing problem is that nothing is known about possible connections between Zwaardemaker's classification and the processes that take place in the brain (rhinencephalon).

Finally we should mention the smell model devised by Henning, in which olfactory impressions are represented in a geometric way.[72] Each smell is depicted as a point in a prism, defined by the axes flowery-spicy, rotten-burnt and fruity-resinous. In practice, however, it turns out to be very difficult to assign each smell a place on one of those axes. Indeed, some researchers are prejudiced against all methods of classification based on olfactory impressions, because they believe that the qualitative assessment of many smells is to a high degree culturally determined.[73] Others challenge that view; from recent research it appears that there are striking similarities in the appreciation of smells among different cultures. We shall return to this point.

Naming Smells

Smells can also be classified according to the terms used by perfumers, among others, to characterize scents. Arctander has written a standard work on the subject.[74] In this book more than two thousand scents used in the cosmetic and food industries are described in terms of familiar flowers, spices, foods, drinks and so forth. In a manner of speaking, you can designate the smell of your beloved by referring to a rose, honey or apricot with a touch of geranium, or, say, amber or civet. The author used almost three hundred different terms for the impressions evoked by the fragrances.

Frequently occurring terms (approximately seventy) were subjected to a factor analysis. This statistical processing technique enables one to check whether there are sets of terms which belong together—that is, concepts which are often used in an interconnected way. If there are only a few large sets that partly overlap, one may say that the notions used express scarcely anything specific. If there are a large number of small groups as well as the necessary isolated designations, one may conclude that the terminology is functioning well—that it actually distinguishes smells. The results of this analysis do not tally with the intuition of people who are accustomed to smelling a great deal and very acutely, and who believe that it is an impossible task to try to distinguish the thousands of smells from each other in a linguistically sound way. The result was that from the 74 frequently occurring terms 27 clusters could be formed, only a few of which contained more than three terms. One such cluster consisted of "pear/banana/pineapple," another of "wax/oil/fat." The elements of the latter do not correspond with those of the cluster "butter/cream," so that statistically there is reason to assume that "fat" expresses a different olfactory quality than "butter." Everyone will be prepared to accept this; a sandwich containing fat smells and tastes differently than one containing butter. Approximately 14 terms, such as almond, tea, caramel, could not be accommodated in any cluster.

This research is important because many of Arctander's terms do not overlap, which suggests that they really do express something about the perceptual qualities of a fragrance. If every olfactory researcher could adopt the terminology and after some training apply it, the search for primary smells might become redundant. Up to now the search for such smells has been dominated by an approach that looks at the chemical qualities or the form of the molecule; however, it is doubtful whether a great deal can be expected from this. Perhaps it might be more sensible to try to describe olfactory *impressions* more closely in what is obviously the quite precise vocabulary of Arctander in order to determine what the essential qualities of different kinds of smells are. If primary smells exist, they probably number no more than a few dozen.

Classification on the Basis of Chemical Structure

Back to the great problem which has still not been solved: what factor or factors are responsible for the qualities of an olfactory sensation? From the standpoint of chemistry, it was believed for some time that the form of the molecule was decisive for the olfactory sensation—that is, a kind of key-lock system.[75] A characteristic of this stereochemical theory is that it is based on two factors, shape and size. It was claimed, for example, that a camphor-like smell was based on round molecules with a cross section of seven angstroms, a musk-like smell was evoked by disk-shaped molecules measuring ten angstroms, wedge-shaped molecules are responsible for the smell of peppermint, and so on. The deviser of this theory originally believed that there were seven primary smells: fish, sperm, sweat, urine, malt, mint and musk; he based this notion on (among other things) specific forms of color blindness. Despite attempts by other researchers to supply additional data, it did not prove possible to explain a reasonable number of olfactory sensations in this way; moreover, the number of "primary smells" soon climbed to thirty—an unmanageable number.[76]

Other researchers, with varying success, attempted to classify smells on the basis of the chemical properties of fragrances. The discovery of smell-binding proteins and the existence of specific types of anosmia, led, as we have seen, to the idea that eventually primary smells would be discovered by analogy with primary colors—and specific forms of color blindness. In this context an extensive study was made of *structure-odor relationships* (SOR),[77] in which a search was conducted for functional chemical compounds or configurations within the molecule which were purportedly essential for the olfactory sensation. An example: We take a simple hydrocarbon chain into which an oxygen atom is built. It is conceivable that the location of this atom is decisive for the nature of the smell. That principle is called regional selectivity: the position of the functional group within a chain determines the smell that is perceived, and small variations in the position of that group can cause a marked difference in the experience of smell.

For example, vanillin is chemically virtually identical to iso-vanillin (an OH and an OCH_3 group have changed position). Vanillin gives flan its specific smell, but iso-vanillin is odorless.

Apart from the possible significance of functional groups, and that of the form and size of the molecule, various other factors may have effects within such an SOR system. First of all, one can think of the position of unsaturated links in the molecule. The smell of unsaturated jasmone, a component of jasmine, has a subtlety lacking in the saturated form. People have also considered the distance between the functional groups within a molecule. If that distance is greater than 0.3 nanometer, the receptor protein can no longer grasp the odor molecule in a sufficient number of places at once, with the result that the odor cannot be smelled. Finally the *chirality* of the molecule may be at issue: molecules which are each other's mirror image may differ considerably in their perceived intensity and quality.[78] For example, androstadinone, one of the male pheromone-like substances, smells somewhat like urine, while the chemical mirror image of this substance is odorless.

To summarize: Data on the link between the structure of a substance and its smell are far from unambiguous; it turns out to be very difficult to find a constant link between the molecular structure and the associated olfactory sensations. One of the few concrete findings is the "triaxial rule." Large molecules—if there is to be an olfactory sensation—must be grasped in at least three places by the receptor protein. If it is grasped in only one or two places, the receptor protein is insufficiently activated, so that there is no olfactory sensation. On the basis of this principle it is understandable that a substance like androstenol evokes a powerful olfactory sensation, while a molecule built from the same atoms (in this case the *three beta-epimer*) is odorless. (In this epimer an H atom is exchanged for an OH group, with the result that the necessary number of points of attachment are no longer in one plane.) Finally, the possible chain *length* of odors may play a part. If people are confronted with a series of simple alcohols (for example, methanol, ethanol, butanol, pentanol) and simple acetates, they are inclined to confuse substances with the same length of chain.[79]

In any case, this kind of research has made it clear that the olfactory sensation is a very complicated—and capricious—process. Indeed some researchers compare the properties of the olfactory organ with those of the physical immune system. The immune system, too, not only is complex but displays many differences within and between people. For example, if a number of people are exposed to the cold virus, as a rule only a relatively small percentage will become ill (principally those who in the few days of exposure had "unpleasant events" to cope with: daily hassles affect the immune system). In the same way, in periods when students work long days preparing for examinations the quality of the immune system falls; after the loss of a loved one or a precious possession it remains below normal for months.

Although research into the connection between perception and the chemical structure of odors is therefore characterized by laborious small steps forward, nevertheless much useful and usable knowledge has been gathered. For example, it is now possible to manufacture artificial smells and tastes. The perfume industry uses much less musk and amber (precious substances of animal origin) than it once did, instead using synthetic substances with appropriate functional groups, such as aldehydes. By experimenting with all kinds of variants, it is possible to repeatedly find new fragrances, which also lead to new or hitherto unknown olfactory impressions. Because of their commercial importance, many of these synthetic substances have been patented and trademarked.

On the basis of chemical structure, then, *something* can be said about which odors belong together and which do not; but in general we are forced to conclude that the sensation of a smell is determined by a large number of other, largely unknown factors. In short, substances that are scarcely similar chemically may evoke virtually the same olfactory impression and vice versa. No molecular or chemical theory can explain these phenomena in a satisfactory way.

The Measuring of Olfactory Sensations

The different qualities of the experience of smell, such as subjective intensity, can be expressed and measured in various ways.

One way is quantitative, via an appreciation scale running from 1 to 10 (magnitude estimation). Another, more qualitative method involves using the terminology of another sense: a smell may be intense, high, warm or sweet.[80] "There is an intense, high, warm and sweet smell here" need not be an absurd statement if intense, high, warm and sweet say something about the intensity or the quality of a sense impression. In practice, of course, it happens differently: in an experiment, one causes the intensity of smells to be registered with the help of an adjustable light source, the level of the sound and suchlike.

It is not easy to investigate the olfactory capacity, even with simple measurements. If one wants to find the link between the concentration of an odor and the intensity of the perception, it is not sensible to simply to hold an odor strip (an impregnated piece of paper) to the nose of a subject at different distances. In order to determine the threshold value—the concentration of an odor that is perceived by at least 50 percent of the section of the population which smells normally—requires refined methods and good dosing equipment. Statistical processing is also essential, because threshold measurements are linked with odd phenomena. For example, people regularly indicate that they can smell something when the concentration of an odor presented is zero (a "false alarm"); conversely they sometimes do not react to a relatively high concentration (a "miss"). So scoring techniques and processing methods that discount these errors must be applied.[81] Erroneous reports may also be based on unintentional mixing of smells: the material of the experimental apparatus may give off a smell; the atmosphere in the laboratory is not always odorless, nor is that of the test subjects in the research area. A relatively inconstant factor is also the passage of air over the olfactory organ, which in practice means that a precisely measured concentration of a substance is not and *cannot* by any means always be smelled in a consistent way.

As has been noted, in the last few decades olfactometers have been devised in order to combat these problems as far as possible. These devices are made of odorless material and the quantity of substance administered can be controlled efficiently. It is even possible to keep the passage of air over the olfactory organ quite constant—for example, with the aid of Teflon tubes in the nostrils. However—in relatively simple qualitative research—vials containing odors and odor strips are sufficient, as has been shown by research into the capacity to name or remember smells.

Although we owe a great deal of knowledge to the olfactometer, we must ask whether this method always imitates reality sufficiently, because when we smell in everyday life we display all variations of sniffing behavior, which is difficult or even impossible to reproduce in experiments with such a device. Research into other senses, such as sight, indicates that *variation* of a stimulus is essential to perception. As far as smell is concerned, variation comes out of a combination of turbulence of the airflow in the nostrils and sniffing. Factors such as the volume of air inhaled in reaction to an olfactory sensation are generally given no account, nor is the lowering of the threshold value through "practice" (see below). Finally, research generally pays little attention to the great intraindividual variation in sensitivity to smells—although this can be established with an olfactometer. In short, this method has its limitations. Much has been learned with the aid of the olfactometer, but certain data are not directly transferable, because in everyday life the sense of smell functions in a way that does not always correspond to the characteristics of this instrument.

In many cases a short stimulus is sufficient to achieve a sensation of smell: a single sniff often leads to the recognition of the smell of almond, eucalyptus or clove. Even if you ask people to inhale the odor in a sniff as short as possible, they are usually able to recognize the smell. The shortest sniff in man lasts approximately 400 milliseconds; a shorter time is not possible because of the technical problems of breathing. Particularly if the concentration of the smell is considerably above the threshold value, such a short sniff is sufficient to perceive the smell; several inhalations are necessary if the concentration is just above it.

Smells also have a bearing on the volume of air that is inhaled.[82] If the concentration of acetic acid is increased, the amount of air investigated by the nose is reduced. This phenomenon is obviously connected with the irritation experienced by the person in smelling. On the other hand, pleasurable smells often lead to an increase in the volume of air inhaled.

Another characteristic of the olfactory organ which does not make research any easier is the fact that the threshold value of fragrances falls the longer the experiment lasts.[83] In other words, if you know a smell, you will need smaller and smaller amounts of the substance in order to recognize it again. This increase in sensitivity, however, has no effect on the threshold values of other fragrances, provided these are not too similar to the substance being tested.

Differences in Sensitivity

It has emerged that the professional noses of perfumers do not perform any better than untrained olfactory organs, certainly when smelling substances they are not familiar with. Nor are professionals any better at identifying smells they know only as well as laymen.[84] Nevertheless, there definitely can be large discrepancies between one person's olfactory organ and another's. The threshold value of limonene (lemon or orange smell), for example, may be no less than 4,000 times higher in one person than in another. There is relatively little variation observable in toluene: a difference of a factor of 5 has been found. It is not known whether such individual differences are connected with a systematic factor, such as the toxicity of a fragrance. From an evolutionary point of view, you might reason that when confronted with dangerous substances the olfactory capacity would display relatively few discrepancies: all people have an interest in detecting such a substance quickly and efficiently, and will not recklessly inhale a high concentration of it. This means that generally the threshold value of dangerous substances must be relatively low. Often that is the case: many of those substances are detected at a moment when they are not yet harmful, but there are exceptions—such as the odorless and deadly carbon monoxide, as well as high concentrations of sulphuric acid.

We can also express the differences in another way. With regard to sensitivity for most smells the rule of thumb is that 96 percent of test subjects score between $\frac{1}{16}$ and 16 times the average. This variation reflects not only differences between people but also differences in the olfactory sensitivity within each individual: threshold values can fluctuate enormously in the same person.[85] It is possible that one day someone may smell a particular substance perfectly well, while on the following day a considerably higher dose is necessary or vice versa. In other words, interindividual differences between threshold values may in part be ascribed to intraindividual variation. In this respect the nose functions very differently than the eye: if the eye were like the nose, you would need a different pair of glasses every day or else you'd see different colors. In psychophysical research on smells this fact is not always taken into account; generally it is assumed that a person's olfactory capacity is relatively stable. The laboriously developed "pure" measuring methods are usable and useful, but in view of the capricious nature of the sense of smell they have their limitations.

It must not be deduced from these remarks that research into threshold values has no significance. Important discoveries have been made. For example, there is a remarkable regularity or order in the threshold values for hydrocarbon chains (alkanoles) such as methanol, ethanol, propanol, butanol and pentanol. As the length of the chain increases, the threshold falls; thus the sensitivity becomes greater the longer or heavier the chain is.[86] For a chain containing eight carbon atoms (octanol) the threshold value is approximately 10 ppb (10 molecules per billion units), and for one carbon atom (methanol) it is 1,000 ppm (1,000 molecules per million units)—which implies an enormous difference. If you convert the threshold value into percentages of saturated steam, then the range is much smaller: from 0.01 percent with a chain of eight atoms to 1 percent for a "chain" with one atom.

People suffering from anosmia for alkanoles can perceive these substances, but they do so through the trigeminal system. In this case a similar regularity occurs. One difference, however, is that the threshold value with the trigeminal system is on average no less than one thousand times higher; measured in percentages of saturated steam the air must contain between 10 and 60 percent hydrocarbon steam. Researchers have tried to map these kinds of relations between structure and operation, in the hope that the psychophysics of smell will not remain stuck in a phase of cataloguing, but will eventually enter an explanatory phase.

Habituation to Smells

We get used to smells very quickly, particularly if they are not alarming or unpleasant. There are countless examples from everyday life. Going into a bakery or bar and grill we are overwhelmed by olfactory impressions, but after we have been there for a while we scarcely perceive the smells anymore. Pet owners' houses sometimes smell of their pets—dogs, cats, guinea pigs—but often the visitor is no longer aware of the smell after a minute or two. In short, the continuing perception of a smell generally leads to a lessening of the perceived intensity. The reverse is also true: if a smell has not been detected for a while, a renewed acquaintance is particularly striking.

This phenomenon (which applies to all the senses) is called adaptation. It implies that sensitivity of a sense is "adjusted" to circumstances—that is, to the duration and intensity of the stimulus. In the case of the eye, sensitivity to light can vary by a factor of ten million (the "adaptation to the dark," however, takes nearly three-quarters of an hour); in the case of hearing, the factor is approximately 100,000. This aspect of the sense of smell has been studied intensively. The direct effect of adaptation can be seen in eating: with a few exceptions, during meals we don't mix everything up together, but take successive mouthfuls of the various foods. Through a variation in the stimulation of smell and taste we achieve an optimum sensation of taste of the food, and in that way the degree of adaptation of both senses is inhibited somewhat.

The sense of smell adapts in two ways. In self-adaptation the sensitivity to a smell depends on how long the smell is smelled and how intense it is; in cross-adaptation the nose's adaptation to a particular smell may affect its sensitivity to another smell. In adaptation experiments, the subject is asked to smell a particular odor for a particular length of time in a particular concentration.

This odor is called the adapting stimulus. After this, the threshold value is established for this substance (self-adaptation) or for another substance (cross-adaptation). It goes without saying that in self-adaptation the threshold value rises the longer the adapting stimulus is allowed to work and the stronger it is. The link between the two is not direct, however, and it varies from substance to substance.[87] If an adapting odor is smelled for a long period, after a certain point the effect on the threshold value for the *adapted* odor is maximized, so a longer exposure to the *adapting* odor does not increase the concentration needed for the subject to recognize the adapted odor. Strong stimuli generally lead to a relatively severe loss in sensitivity; on the other hand, sensitivity is restored most quickly during the first few minutes (a phenomenon that applies to various other senses). So there is a snag in the process of adaptation. This may mean that two different mechanisms are involved—there might be a rapidly operating central process in the brain and a much slower change in the olfactory organ itself (or vice versa)—but that need not be the case. The adaptation curve of the eye to the dark also displays a snag, but this is caused by the different adaptation and recovery speeds of two groups of light-sensitive cells in the retina—the rods and the cones.

Research into adaptation and cross-adaptation aims not only to find out more about the operation of the olfactory organ and the rhinencephalon but also to explore differences and correspondences between fragrances.[88] Since one substance tempers the perception of another, there is reason to assume that these substances are processed in a similar way by the olfactory organ, although they differ chemically. If cross-adaptation is almost as strong as self-adaptation, the same receptors may be involved in the perception of the substance concerned, and the similarity between the smells may be considerable. Unfortunately, the data in this area are far from unambiguous. There follow a few brief findings, which are somewhat controversial.

The effect of odor A on the perception of odor B is in many cases very different than the effect of odor B on the perception of odor A; most cross-adaptive relations are not symmetrical. Moreover, it is possible that one substance may adapt the perception of another substance more strongly than it does itself; in that case cross-adaptation is more pronounced than self-adaptation. Finally, very occasionally in the case of cross-adaptation there seems to be facilitation or intensification: the confrontation with a particular smell *improves* the sensitivity to another substance. In that case, too, research is in the phase of cataloguing, and for the time being little is understood of the observed phenomena. Indeed it is still largely unclear what mechanisms are responsible for (self-) adaptation. Both at the peripheral level (the sensory cells) and at the central level (the rhinencephalon) there are countless factors that affect the perception of smell. In the olfactory organ itself the odor-binding proteins in the membranes of the sensory cells require a certain time to recover after having been in contact with a fragrance. The sensory cells themselves cannot sustain an increased electrified activity for very long. After a discharge they have to build a resting potential again by pumping out ions. These chemical processes take place so quickly, however, that adaptation cannot be explained in that way. Continuing stimulation by a single smell does have a somewhat retarding effect on various chemical processes in the sensory cells, but even when adaptation occurs, a number of smell receptors continue to operate normally. This has been shown by the following experiment.[89]

For a few seconds a cloth impregnated with a certain mixture of smells (heptanol and amyl acetate) is held in front of the nose of a sleeping child. The child subsequently becomes restless and his breathing rhythm changes, but if the smell is not too strong, the child simply continues sleeping. After half a minute the action is repeated; the strength of the reaction decreases. After still more repetitions the child will at a certain point no longer react at all. If this were a case of general tiredness and exhaustion at the level of chemical processes within the sensory cells, one might expect that the child would subsequently show no reaction to one of the components of the mixture. This is not the case, however: if the cloth contains only amyl acetate, the child again reacts as though a new stimulus were being applied.

Another question is whether stimulation of one nostril affects the perception of smell and the state of adaptation of the olfactory

organ on the other side. In one experiment, the test subject inhaled a stimulus at quite a high concentration, after which the
degree of adaptation was measured. The same was done on the
basis of varying, much lower concentrations. In the experiment
proper a number of combinations of two stimuli—namely, the
powerful stimulus and one of the weak stimuli—was applied in
one inhalation to *both* nostrils, so that as far as possible the stimulus on one side was prevented from significantly influencing the
olfactory organ on the other side via the nasopharynx (the connection between the nasal and throat cavities). Subsequently the
state of adaptation of the separate olfactory organs was determined; if they have no effect on each other there should be a
great difference in their loss of sensitivity. That appeared to be
only partly the case: the strongly stimulated olfactory organ was
more highly adapted than the other organ, but a not insubstantial
percentage of the loss of sensitivity of one organ was ascribable
to adaptation of the other. In short, a strongly stimulated olfactory
organ influences its weakly stimulated neighbor (and to a certain
extent vice versa). These data have also been found for other substances, which means that the two olfactory organs influence each
other.[90]

The olfactory bulbi, where smell signals enter, are responsible
for such connections. If these are able to communicate efficiently
with each other, the activity of one olfactory organ has consequences for the sensitivity of the other. Research in rats has shown
that the phenomenon just described is canceled to a large extent
when the foremost cross-connection between the halves of the
brain (*commissura anterior*) is severed.

But this is not the end of the story: the olfactory organs also
affect each other because of the architecture of the nasal and
throat cavities. This was shown as follows: In a rat one olfactory
bulbus was removed surgically, and the nostril on the other side
was blocked. If such an animal is subsequently allowed to smell
through the remaining nostril, it retains some ability to perceive
smells.[91] This can have no other explanation than that the fragrance reaches the undamaged olfactory organ via the nasopharynx, which is also plausible.

However, we must beware of regarding a perceptible change

in behavior as an effect of adaptation, and of assuming that perception does not penetrate at all. There are indications that fragrances which are not smelled (because of adaptation or for some other reason, such as anosmia) may have an effect on the electrical resistance of the skin. In some way or other the information is processed in the "autonomous" nervous system.

Though many aspects of the adaptation process have not yet been clarified, it is believed to take place both in the olfactory organ and in "various levels" in the brain.[92] Perhaps adaptation should be seen not only as a weakening of the reaction of the sensory cells in the nose due to exhaustion; a loss of sensitivity to smells is also connected with habituation, or "boredom" at the level of the brain. The olfactory signals are finally ignored, although they come in almost as clearly and vividly as in the initial phase of the stimulus. The substances concerned are consciously perceived again only if there is a change in their composition or if the subject concentrates on the smell. In this respect smell can be compared with hearing: in the long run you are no longer aware of the ticking of the clock, but you hear the sound again when someone asks what time it is or if you have to pay attention to the time because of an appointment.

To summarize: adaptation and habituation are difficult to distinguish in the case of smell because the olfactory organs communicate with each other in various ways, via the nasopharynx and via cross-connections in the brain. That problem does not arise with all species of animals: in the case of the crab, habituation is exclusively a characteristic of the olfactory organ itself. A research into the adaptation in the chemoreceptor cells in the crab *Homarus americanus* shows that an important function of the sensory system resides in reaction to *changes* in the intensity of the stimulus.[93] This creature has receptors in its claws that can detect ammonia compounds. These cells react not so much to the strength of the concentration as to changes in it. If the concentration of ammonium chloride (sal ammoniac) is very gradually increased, the sensory cells gradually begin to "fire" as frequently as in the resting state. In the case of the frog, one can see something similar in the reaction to differences in temperature. If you put a frog into a pan of warm water, it will try to escape, but if you slowly warm the water, the frog notices nothing and allows itself to be boiled to death.

Quantity Affects Quality

In all the senses a change in the quantitative properties of the stimulus also has consequences for the psychological characteristics of the associated perception. In the field of sight, for example, we are familiar with the *Bezold-Brücke phenomenon*: a slight variation in a perceived color, although the wavelength remains the same, as the intensity of light is changed. By analogy, in hearing there are variations in the perceived pitch when the volume varies (the *Zürmühl-Stevens effect*). From this it appears that senses are not rigid or "objective" registration instruments. They are biological systems which — in interaction with the relevant parts of the brain — not only gather information but also give it a different form or meaning.

This principle also applies to smell. Depending on the concentration, a single smell can cause diverse olfactory sensations. Many substances are characterized by a twofold (or even threefold) effect, which means that there are different impressions with different quantities.[94] As a rule of thumb one can say that many substances which cause a stench not only stink less as the concentration decreases but gradually even begin to smell *pleasant*. As yet there is no explanation for this phenomenon.

Some examples of such a turnaround in appreciation with a change in the concentration of fragrances are the following: The perfume industry makes frequent use of indole, a compound that forms the basis of skatole, the substance that makes feces stink. In low concentrations, however, indole smells of flowers. If the rather aggressively smelling thiol (tetrahydrothiophene), which is added to natural gas, is diluted considerably, it starts to smell like coffee. Civet, the glandular secretion produced by the sexual organs of civet cats, smells penetrating and unpleasant in high concentrations, but in low concentrations it has a wonderful smell — the reason why it is prized in the Far East. Amber derives from the intestines of the whale. It is probably rotting or pathological tissue (cancer) which floats in the sea in lumps. In the past little balls were made of it (pomanders). These were worn on a necklace to prevent diseases such as the plague and even as an aphrodisiac.[95] Heptanol, which in high concentrations has a suffocating smell, is used in small quantities in perfume and smells very pleasant. Ozone irritates the breathing passages and dissolved in air is even poisonous if the quantity is large (as during rush hour on a warm, windless day), but in low concentrations it smells fresh and pleasant.

In short, many notorious stenches not only begin to smell less unpleasant at low intensities but may even give off a pleasant smell. There are also exceptions to this rule. Camphor, for example, has an aromatic, woody smell, which as it is diluted has a smell more and more similar to the smell of urine. In small quantities, toxic sulphuric acid smells like rotten eggs, but in a high dosage the substance becomes odorless—and dangerous. In oil refineries sulphuric acid may be released in high concentrations; as a result, many people have lost their lives.[96]

Another rule is that you must use a pleasant smell with moderation. At a high intensity, the trigeminal nerve in the face often becomes irritated, which is counterproductive for the experience of smell. The external nose doesn't hurt, but breathing in through the nose becomes unpleasant—the eyes start watering, the cheeks contract. Usually there is a switch to breathing through the mouth and one takes a few steps back or in a different direction until the stimulus is discontinued. In one common instance, small children who like the smell of flowers and who may perhaps not yet have a fully developed trigeminal system tend to be wasteful with toilet spray.[97] Perhaps such a spray has a less suffocating effect for a child, and the child finds the smell pleasant even in high concentrations. The function of the spray can in the toilet is not based on the principle of smelling "something else": if fragrances are mixed in very *unequal* quantities, one smell more or less obscures the other.

Smell Pollution and Mixtures

The aroma of freshly made coffee and tea or toast with melted butter and cheese on it is generally found to be pleasant, even in combination with aftershave and perfume; the stench of a chemical plant and the smell of cars tearing along the roads are unpleasant. Almost all pleasant everyday smells (despite their great differences) have one characteristic in common: they are not pure odors, but mixtures.

One of the countless problems associated with traditional smell research is that generally pure fragrances are used, whereas in nature these occur never or rarely. Odors are almost always impure; they are virtually always parts of mixtures with many ingredients, all of which make specific contributions to the mixture. For example, the aroma of coffee, cognac, orange peel and roasted meat are composed of many hundreds of substances, and the disgusting "cocktail" found in office buildings may even consist of more than a thousand substances (tobacco smoke, body odors, perfumes, emissions from floor covering, inadequately filtered air). In a certain sense the nose itself also mixes odors, because we have two olfactory organs. Nevertheless, we do not have the impression that our perception of smell is "split," just as we are generally not aware in seeing and hearing that we have two eyes and two ears.

The perceived intensity of a mixture is almost never the sum of the intensity of the constituent parts. This fact is of particular importance in combating smell pollution. A stench is rarely caused by a single substance in a mixture; interaction between various substances is much more important. In addition, it is possible that a foul-smelling mixture may stink even worse if one removes one of the culprits: substances may compensate for or neutralize each other's stink. In principle it may be possible to combat stench with stench: one stench-causing substance may neutralize the effect of another, provided the concentrations are *unequal*. To make matters worse, it is possible that the stink of a mixture may become worse when a well-meaning chemist adds a *pleasant* odor to the whole, and even substances that are themselves odorless may contribute to the subjective properties of the whole. The perceived intensity of a mixture therefore shows a number of strange discrepancies and is rarely predictable.

Statistical examples indicate the kinds of things that can happen. In mixing two odors, a (fictive intensity 5) and b (intensity 7), the following results are possible: summation (ab = 12), partial summation (e.g., ab = 10), a compromise (ab = 6), neutralization or partial obscuring (ab = 0 or another number lower than 5) and reinforcement or synergy (such as ab = 15). In many cases the intensity of a mixture is a partial sum of the intensity of the constituents. For those phenomena a mathematical model has been developed, which turns out also to apply in determining the general impression made by smell and taste.[98]

One can say that a sum and synergy are found particularly in low concentrations of fragrances. For example, the intensity of a mixture of pyridine (a substance added to spirits) and rotten eggs is synergetic even in small quantities. However, compromises and neutralization are found to occur in higher concentrations and with a very *unequal* mixture.

Some researchers assume that the smells of a mixture are perceived by the same group of receptors in the olfactory organ.[99] If in a high concentration the capacity of the sensory cells involved is used to its maximum, a problem will arise in still higher concentrations, because the substances will have to "compete" with each other in order to be able to link with the receptor proteins. In theory this phenomenon may lead to a compromise or even to the obscuring of smells. This explanation is only partly adequate, however. A lemon smell masks the smell of vinegar provided the concentration is high enough. The reverse is not the case; the smell of vinegar is not capable of dispelling a lemon smell. Many masking effects are asymmetrical. Why this is so is not known in all cases, but in a few cases we do know why.

Experiments have been conducted in which people have been asked to smell vials containing one substance in ever-increasing concentrations. The subjects were asked to pause after each sniff, to cancel out the olfactory system's loss of sensitivity. They were asked to indicate the perceived intensity of the vials. They estimated the strength from case to case; the link between the concentration and the subjective intensity can be calculated and presented graphically with a "rising function" (generally an exponential one). In the case of single alcohols, propanol and dodecanol have approximately the same rising function. In the case of heptanol, however, the perceived intensity rises much less rapidly when there is a proportional rise in quantity. Suppose we mix propanol and heptanol. That mixture gives rise to a particular olfactory sensation. If we dilute the mixture as part of an attempt to combat the stink, the smell of heptanol becomes relatively stronger, which may mean that the action has not so great an effect. There is the further problem that the nose adapts to one substance much more quickly than to another. Habituation to propanol occurs much faster than habituation to naphthalene. If the two substances form a mixture, after a time we therefore smell only naphthalene.[100]

Thus it is very difficult to give general guidelines on combating a stench. Sometimes it will be a question of trial and error, unless one knows the speed of adaptation and the rising functions of all the substances involved. Generally that knowledge does not exist. Industries would therefore be wiser if they tackled the sources of a stench itself as far as possible, instead of masking it with other odors. The careless accumulation of all kinds of masking smells may provoke new problems: if there are different speeds of adaptation, the stench will be smelled again shortly afterward.

In addition, it is possible to rid areas of smells through oxidation aids such as hydrogen peroxide and chlorine, or with absorbents based on silica gel, aluminium hydroxide or china clay. A disadvantage of these substances is that they can dispel both unpleasant and pleasant smells. An alternative is the following: Bacteria can break down organic material and convert it into natural gas. That process, however, releases stinking and toxic sulphuric acid. This substance can be neutralized with caustic soda, but that substance is harmful to the environment. A provisional solution involves allowing the bacteria to break down most of the sulphuric acid, after which a little caustic soda can do the rest. A few purification plants use this technique.

A final problem in this connection: As the concentration of odors increases, the trigeminal system becomes more and more irritated. Chlorine (to mention an extreme example) dispels all kinds of smells, but is literally breathtaking. Air fresheners are particularly useful when there is a touch of stench, such as in the toilet, which eventually would go away even without a freshener. And the best way of dispelling the smell of cat litter is to keep the box clean. In olfactometers, activated charcoal is used to purify the air before it is mixed with a fragrance.[101] But charcoal filters all smells, hence also harmless or pleasant smells. Moreover, it is quite expensive to use charcoal on a large scale to combat stench.

A form of smell pollution can also occur with cheap perfumes. Many of those fragrances consist of mixtures of substances which evaporate at different rates and/or have different speeds of adaptation. The results can be dramatic: the mixture smells nice at first but after a while begins to stink; or a perfume may smell different on one person than on another due to the mixture with body odor, chemical reactions which are found on the skin and suchlike.

Analyzing and Identifying Mixtures

The olfactory organ can distinguish several hundred thousand odors, provided they are presented separately. Note that distinguishing is different from recognizing or naming. Distinguishing trans-2-hexanol (a fruity smell) and trans-2-decanol (a rancid smell) is not difficult, even though you don't know what substances are involved.[102] But what happens if hexanol is mixed with decanol? How efficiently can the nose identify different components in a mixture? In this respect the olfactory organ does not perform very well. It has been observed that mixtures of two known and familiar smells (examples of substances used included camphor, lemon, almond, vinegar and peppermint) were correctly identified by only 12 percent of test subjects.[103] In mixtures of five smells this percentage fell to zero. Professional smellers like perfumers perform scarcely any better: only 3 percent of them were able to identify all the constituents of a five-part mixture. It is also striking that mixtures of three or more components are assessed as just as complicated or equally "unidentifiable." Unpleasant smells, however, are generally better spotted and recognized in a mixture than pleasant ones. In the case of a mixture the olfactory organ focuses first on one smell: no less than 80 percent of test subjects are generally able to identify one decidedly unpleasant-smelling substance in a mixture. The dominance of a particular smell in a mixture may be connected with the fact that the recognition of smells goes hand in hand with different reaction times. The "suppressed" substances may need more time to be recognized, so the substance that makes the first impression determines our assessment of the mixture as a whole. But this reasoning is open to doubt; the reaction times may differ, but they do not predict what substances have preference in identification.[104]

Do these smells in a mixture confuse us because we do not know what to pay attention to? Would we be more successful if we were asked to focus our attention on a particular constituent? This possibility has been investigated by asking test subjects to concentrate on the smell of almond during the first week of an experiment and to report when this was in a mixture; the second week it was peppermint's turn, the third week orange's, and so on.[105] There was a slight improvement in performance, but generally the results were not very encouraging. Obviously the olfactory organ finds it hard to analyze mixtures. Even if you present two perfume bottles with the same mixtures, in many cases they are perceived differently. The reverse happens even more often: if you leave one component out of a mixture of three components (for example, linalool, sineol and carvone), over one-third of test subjects believe that the samples do not differ or scarcely differ.[106] In short, mixtures normally smell like a single odor.

Nevertheless, we must not underestimate the nose's analytical capacities. A number of things are simply not known in this area, because the research methods used are not always appropriate; people are asked, for example, to identify *constituents*, not the general impression of a mixture. For that reason, smell profiles have been made of various substances using a list of 152 descriptions (such as grassy, aromatic, fruity, rancid, soapy, sharp, stinking).[107] This was also done for mixtures consisting of various concentrations of diverse components. Such a smell profile can be regarded as a frequency distribution of descriptions which the test subjects give to a smell; by comparing smell profiles, you can say something about the degree of equivalence in the impression made by the smells. The results show that we are definitely capable of recognizing certain constituents in mixtures. One rule is the following: as the concentration of one of the ingredients increases, the profile of the mixture as a whole becomes more and more similar to the characteristics of *that* substance. Often there turns out to be a sharp transition from one profile to another, which means that another component becomes dominant in perception. If research methods take greater account of the normal daily practice of identifying and analyzing smells and mixtures, we seem to have more to offer: there are circumstances under which components of a mixture are recognized.

There is something dishonest about this discussion, though: the same problem occurs with the other senses. Only people who are highly trained musically are capable of analyzing a five-note chord struck on a piano; we only know from school that purple is a mixture of blue and red, and most people are not capable of disentangling a mixture of sweet, salty, sour and bitter (the basic tastes).

A Half-Blocked Nose

Sometimes both nasal canals are blocked, but usually only one of the two is. We are seldom able to breathe freely through both nostrils at once. The process varies rhythmically. The background of this odd phenomenon is not known. We mentioned the hypothesis that mankind went through a "water ape period." One of our ancestors was supposed to have fed on sea creatures and plants while wading and diving. Like other diving mammals, it is theorized, it possessed a muscle that enabled it to close its nostrils before taking to the water.[108] Perhaps the alternating passability of the nasal cavities is based on the rudimentary remnant of that muscle, but this does not explain why the process is rhythmic.

Another possibility is that the periodic alternation is necessary in order to limit harmful effects from outside. While one nasal canal is free, passable and "on duty," the other can rest and the mucous layer has an opportunity to recover.[109]

A phenomenon obscurely connected with this is that the activity of both hemispheres of the brain more or less follows the passability of the nasal canals. When the right nasal canal is open, the left half of the brain is relatively active, and vice versa. No explanation has been found for this. Most connections between the body and the brain are crossed, but that does not apply to connections between the brain and the olfactory organs. Probably this phenomenon is not caused by a need to grasp smells in a special way in the brain; rather, it may be related to one of the many odd "behavioral remnants" from earlier times which still determine our functioning and which are not easily explained.[110] Finally, it is asserted that forced breathing through one nostril can activate the opposite half of the brain, a method used in the treatment of mild depressions (namely, intensive breathing through only the left nostril; how that is supposed to work, no one understands).[111]

Smelling Direction

The nose has not only two entries but also two olfactory organs. Biologists like to posit a functional basis for the fact that various organs in our body occur in pairs. A reserve organ is very useful, particularly if the system is sensitive to damage or defects. However, this is not a generally applicable principle. We have only one heart, stomach, liver, pancreas, etc. A biological-evolutionary mechanism of cell division probably led through chance to the formation of a number of paired organs.

Whatever the reason, man possesses two olfactory organs, as he has two eyes and ears. A double sensory organ can receive more information than a single organ. In the case of all senses present in duplicate there is intensive cooperation. We need both eyes to have a good perception of depth, two ears to locate a source of sound. Is there such a type of cooperation in the case of smell, too? The location and direction of a source of smell can usually be discovered by focusing on the intensity of the smell stimuli, but are there also indications that human beings have a certain capacity for "smell direction" in the true sense?[112]

Let us focus on an experiment to solve this issue. One inserts Teflon tubes into both nostrils, ensuring a constant supply of air. Next, through either the left-hand or the right-hand tube an odor is administered; the test subject is required to indicate which side received the odor. The results are far from unambiguous: some smells are located correctly, others not. In the case of carbon dioxide, there were only 2 wrong responses to 985 presentations; in the case of menthol, 9 out of 913. With vanilla and sulphuric acid (the smell of rotten eggs), the picture was totally different: vanilla scored 394 incorrect responses from 824 presentations, sulphuric acid 441 from 855. So for them it mattered very little on what side the odors were administered.

How is one to explain those differences? As we saw in Chapter 2, some odors are smelled not only through the nose but also through the trigeminal nerve. Carbon dioxide and menthol can activate this nerve. When the trigeminal nerve is stimulated on one side, the information (about direction) will not be lost when it is processed by the brain. That has a purpose, because the trigeminal nerve reacts mainly to aggressive substances which have to be avoided (this would be problematical if you could determine the direction of the source). The questions remain why this is not a generally applicable principle (sulphuric acid is also toxic) and why the olfactory organ does not have the capacity to locate the direction of *all* substances. Locating a source of smell offers a better chance of escaping danger, finding food and so forth. The fact that we are to some extent able to smell direction might be linked with the fact that odors affect mainly the right side of the brain, an area which is important for spatial orientation in general.

In theory the difference in the time of arrival in the left-hand and right-hand olfactory organs may be important, too. The recognition times of smells vary considerably, and a smell impression is not a photo, but a phenomenon embedded in time, comparable to a section of film.[113] Time difference does indeed play a certain part, together with a difference in the intensity of the stimulus. A strongly stimulated nostril affects the sensitivity of the other, and some information about direction is gained.[114]

One of the shortcomings of much of the research which has been outlined is that the fragrances are administered through a constant stream of air, and that they are conducted generally to only one nostril. If one organ perceives nothing and the other does, it is possible that the message is incorrectly interpreted. In daily life, head movements and continual sniffing, as everyone knows, are useful in locating the source of a smell through noticing small differences in intensity, but these kinds of behavior generally play no part in many of the experiments. Future research will therefore have to show to what extent and in what way the olfactory sense manages to determine the direction of the source of a smell. In any case, it will be desirable if laboratory experiments take more account of the natural process of smelling and sniffing.

Chapter 4

Smell Over One's Lifetime

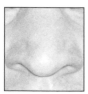ike the other senses, the sense of smell opens up a portion of reality surrounding us. This does not happen in a particularly objective or rational way: as in sight and hearing, the sense of smell adapts and selects the incoming information, and many physiological processes—including our physical desires and needs—affect the experience of smell (the way someone who is hungry is inclined to see steaks in vague pictures). The olfactory organ is linked to the functioning of the organism as a whole; at the same time the genetic "blueprint" probably plays a role, as do habits like smoking and snorting cocaine and many factors that are outside our control in society and the culture at large.

In this chapter we shall deal with the development of the sense of smell through life, the consequences of growing older for the functioning of this sense, the extent to which the capacity to smell in a woman differs from that in a man, and the effects of smoking, occupation, environment and culture on smell.

Smells in the Womb

As discussed in Chapters 1 and 2, probably the first sensory perception in our existence, even before our birth, is of a smell contained in the amniotic fluid.[115] That perception probably does not take place in the olfactory organ, but in the vomeronasal organ, which is formed between the fifth and eighth week of pregnancy. In a later embryonic phase the nerve connections between this organ and the brain degenerate. In adults the cavity in which this organ was situated is sometimes still present, but it contains no more sensory cells, or those cells no longer function.

There are olfactory cells equipped with olfactory cilia on the olfactory epithelium of the human fetus as early as the ninth week. A month later the olfactory bulbi are also formed, and the number of (brain) cells that can process the signals of the sensory cells increases considerably. The trigeminal system also develops rapidly; after about three months it is more or less operational. At a rough estimate, we can say that the unborn child can smell from the fifth month onward. Moreover, it is not inconceivable that smells dissolved in the amniotic fluid fix impressions vital to the fetus's physiological and psychological development. Smell may also create memory associations that after birth will have some importance for mental development and for the bonding process with the mother. Of course, other sensory systems also play a part before birth, particularly hearing (embryos react to a loud noise by moving).

Animal experiments have proved informative in this connection. The smell of amniotic fluid in rats influences the recognition of the mother by her young.[116] This has been shown in the following way. The amniotic fluid of a number of females was gathered during pregnancy in a minor operation conducted with the aid of a microscope. Eight hours after birth young rats were put on a plate, to which a little bud of cotton wool was clipped at the height of one centimeter on the left and right. The bud on one side was moistened with the amniotic fluid of the mother, the bud on the other with the fluid of a non-related female rat. The young invariably sought to approach the bud with their mother's amniotic fluid on it; they moved their heads in that direction and sometimes tried to suck the bud.[117]

In order to exclude the contact between the mother and the young after birth as a possible cause of this behavior, the experiment was also conducted with rats born through caesarean section. These rats were washed and dried and put on the plate with the cotton wool buds. In this case, too, the young rats preferred the bud containing their mother's amniotic fluid. We can therefore conclude that the olfactory organ in these creatures functions before birth and that in that time a primitive "smell memory" develops. Human babies also recognize and prefer the smell of their mother, particularly that of her breasts, armpits and neck, and certain smells can trigger certain behaviors immediately after birth.

Smell in Children

Babies have a preference for certain smells at a very early stage.[118] If you hold odor strips bearing the scent of rotten eggs up to the noses of infants, the infants will turn up their noses and contort their faces as if to cry, while the smell of butter provokes sucking movements. It does not follow from this, however, that babies have an innate aversion to rotten eggs. Possibly the smell of butter resembles the familiar and safe smell of their mother. If their mothers were to smell of rotten eggs, then infants might make sucking movements in response to that unpleasant smell.[119] Possibly babies learn to appreciate or dislike certain smells very quickly, but other smells, such as vanilla, banana and shrimp, which we may assume the baby is smelling for the first time, provoke specific reactions. Obviously the baby's nose quickly makes associations and has a preference for what is familiar; at the same time there seems to be a certain innate appreciation of certain smells. From puberty onward the hedonic order of smells remains relatively constant.

But first something about smell in very young children. In one series of experiments, children from one to five years of age were allowed to play at a table with a screen set up on one side of it.[120] Through openings in the screen, a researcher blew odors toward the table in concentrations far above the threshold value. Judging by the facial expressions of the children, there was no clear evidence that the various age groups preferred particular odors, and half the odors provoked no reaction at all, which leads to the supposition that small children are generally either tolerant of smells or relatively indifferent to them.

Various experiments have shown that from a certain age onward there is a clear change in the appreciation of smells. However, this metamorphosis is connected with the way in which questions are asked and with the cognitive capacity of the child. The older children get, the better they understand the how and why of a test and the more "honest" their answers will be, although some inconsistencies remain. In view of this kind of problem, various different methods have been developed to investigate smell in children. For example, a child is asked to choose a favorite cuddly toy (say, one from *Sesame Street*). Then the child is asked to smell two different odors and say which smell belongs to a pleasant character and which to a character regarded as "unpleasant."[121] In this way you can find out indirectly what a child thinks is nice and what it does not, and from this the hedonic order of smells can be determined. Research with babies and toddlers, for example, can identify no clear break in the experience of smell.[122] If there is a turnaround in a child's appreciation of smells, it happens during puberty, because of the production of sex hormones. During puberty young people suddenly find pleasant odors they once disliked (including pheromone-like substances such as androsterone and musk) and reject substances they once enjoyed (such as vanilla and strawberry). It is also striking that lavender becomes a favorite smell for many people between the ages of sixteen and twenty.

Adults

After the age of twenty the hedonic order and the appreciation of smells remain more or less the same. Tetrahydrothiophene (thiol), the alarm smell of natural gas, is an exception to this rule: this substance is considered less and less unpleasant with the passing of the years.[123] In general, during the first twenty years of life individual fluctuations occur in the appreciation of most smells, but the similarity *within* age groups is strikingly great. The scale of appreciation on which smells are placed also has a much smaller range with toddlers and teenagers than with adults. In other words, as people grow older their responses to smells grow more subjective and richer in associations, until in old age a certain numbing or narrowing occurs.[124] For example, the smell of diesel oil is experienced as much less unpleasant by older people than by younger people.

There is no satisfactory explanation for these phenomena and changes. According to some researchers, in the process of perception different kinds of odors are processed independently of one another.[125] They claim that there is an "intrinsic order" in smelling: smells are decoded in certain perceptual channels, and the corresponding "wiring" constitutes the "hardware" that contains the basic principles of the whole olfactory process. This view would explain limited anosmia, or smell blindness, as a partial defect in the system affecting only the capacity to perceive certain smells; the appreciation of other smells is not at issue. It follows that people who are anosmic for certain substances must have the same judgments as "normal" people, when they are confronted with odors that they can smell. Possibly certain similar smell profiles may be connected to specific receptors, "wiring systems" and areas in the brain.

Older People

Age brings inevitable ailments, Cicero's words of praise to aging notwithstanding.[126] However, this does not mean that young people should smell particularly well. The sense of smell has to mature, and according to most researchers the sensitivity of this sense comes to full bloom only between the ages of thirty and forty. As one grows older, in many cases one becomes wiser, too, which means that certain smells will grow richer in associations. But however experienced and acute one's sense of smell has been, in old age the capacity to name, recognize, distinguish and, finally, smell odors gradually declines and disappears altogether.

The capacity to smell remains reasonably stable in most people until the ages of fifty to sixty: it has been said that the greatest olfactory sensitivity is found in those in their thirties.[127] In older people the loss of smell occurs gradually, as a loss of sensitivity to the whole range of smells. Characteristically, the loss occurs so slowly that the person involved usually notices nothing.[128] One believes that one can still smell and taste well, but experiments show clear evidence of decline. In general, older people are quite content with the taste of food, for example; if they have complaints about food, other reasons are involved, such as poor digestion, limited resources which keep them from buying the foods they need or like, or even the poor quality of groceries compared with those of the past (such as a dislike of the preservatives used today).

The process of decline continues particularly after retirement; the same applies to the other senses. Both the absolute and the relative sensitivity to smells decreases, many threshold values are no less than a hundred times higher in older people than in students, recognizing smells becomes harder and harder and it takes longer and longer for the olfactory system to recover after smelling a strong odor. The aging process of the sense of smell is distinguished by the following physical and physiological changes.

- Nasal cavity problems, such as frequent or chronic viral infections.
- Drying out of the mucous layer (older people have up to 7 percent less bodily fluid), inflammation of the mucous membrane, formation of polyps, poor circulation.[129]
- Calcification of the ethmoid bone; often scar tissue is produced, which obstructs or even blocks the nerve connections running through the perforated ethmoid bone to the rhinencephalon.
- Reduction in the production of new sensory cells.
- Reduction in size of the olfactory organ; the sensory epithelium is replaced by the epithelium of the nasal cavity.
- A sharp drop in the number of sensory cells in the olfactory bulbi.

• Degeneration of the olfactory cortex, which generally also applies to other parts of the brain.

As a result of these changes, three-quarters of people over the age of eighty are anosmic or virtually anosmic, as are half of people between sixty-five and eighty, regardless of conditions of life or culture.[130] In the United States, hundreds of gas explosions occur every year because older people, their sense of smell weakened, either do not notice leaks or notice them much too late. Many older people also fall victim to toxic smoke and fire, when they don't notice food burning, etc. Because smell *and* taste function relatively poorly in older people, they run a greater risk of eating food that has spoiled. In view of the aging population and the increasing isolation of older people, these problems will only grow greater in the future. By way of a consolation, it has been shown that, to the extent that they can still smell and taste, older people can experience the *combined* intensity of smells and tastes more or less as strongly as younger people. Only when smell functions significantly worse than taste, or vice versa, do things go wrong.[131] In other words, a reduced sensitivity of one sense does not always have only unpleasant consequences; the main thing is that smell and taste should remain "in step." Unlike smell, taste generally continues to function reasonably well to an advanced age.[132]

What is one to do? Chemical additives might offer a solution.[133] In one experiment, people who generally complained about the tastelessness of food were asked to choose between "ordinary" food and food treated with artificial odors and taste additives; they preferred the latter, whereas people with an efficiently functioning olfactory organ generally found the treated foods "much too strong" or "too spicy." So it might be a good idea to market "pepped-up" groceries for older people and other people who smell poorly. Adding lots of sugar or salt is not a good idea, of course: what is gained in taste is risked in health and diet. One should be aware of how harmful these substances might be, but if the results are positive, there is no reason to advise older people against them.[134] Good food is necessary; alarming reports have appeared about the malnutrition of people (particularly elderly people) in hospitals, institutions for the elderly and nursing homes. Moreover, one can also improve the taste (and to some extent the smell) of food by adding substances which stimulate the trigeminal nerve.

Smokers, Environment and Work

The olfactory capacity of smokers is generally worse than that of non-smokers. We have to be careful in interpreting this fact: if a smoker is tested shortly after he has put out his cigarette, he smells less because of adaptation to the smoke. According to various researchers, however, there is also a question of direct damage. They claim that the severity of this depends on how long a person has smoked and the amount of tobacco one has consumed. Heavy smokers who have stopped, they assert, have a diminished sense of smell months or even years later.[135] However, it has been shown that the effects of smoking on smell are less severe than those of aging and sex differences.

Nicotine belongs to the alkaloid family, which comprises substances with a strong physiological effect. Other alkaloids are morphine, heroin and cocaine; quinine (used in treating malaria), quinidine (for certain heart diseases) and reserpine (used as a sedative and to reduce blood pressure) are useful medicines. Alkaloids are well known for their addictive and narcotic effects; in addition, the olfactory capacity can experience both acute and chronic disturbance from such substances.[136] The acute effects include blockages or inhibitions of the flow of air in the nose, disruptions of the circulation in the mucous membrane and problems in the signal transfer of nerve impulses. Some disruptions of smell can be traced back to interrupted breathing through the nose; prednisone, a corticosteroid, can normalize breathing through the nose, offering a solution in these cases.

Various other substances have directly harmful effects on our sense of smell. These include not only volatile substances like sulphuric acid, acetone, ammonia, benzene, carbon monoxide and formaldehyde, but also metals such as lead, silver, chromium, mercury and cadmium.[137] People who work a great deal with deter-

Concentration of paint solvent	UPSIT test scores	
	Non-smokers	Smokers
68	35.3	34.5
68–170	33.8	34.6
171 and over	31.1	34.8

gents and solvents (such as paint thinners and the glue once used by hat makers), score lower than others in smell tests. Painters smell significantly worse than their peers in other fields, probably because they inhale solvents in paint as they work.[138]

The following table presents a number of data on the connection between exposure to various concentrations of solvents (indicated in parts per million, or ppm) and the quality of the olfactory sense. Painters who smoke appear to suffer slightly less from loss of smell than their non-smoking colleagues; probably the nicotine in tobacco smoke masks and neutralizes the harmful effects of the solvents and tempers their stupefying effects. (Nicotine to a large extent determines the smell of tobacco smoke: low-nicotine cigarettes stink worse than ordinary ones; they smell somewhat like scorched hay.) Nicotine can mask the smell of other substances; the olfactory epithelium of rats and mice is activated by nicotine.[139]

By mixing a spray containing nicotine with other substances and comparing the resulting EOGs (electro-olfactograms), one can gain some insight into the way in which the sense of smell reacts to such mixtures. It appears that there are specific receptors in the olfactory epithelium that react mainly to substances like nicotine. Therefore it is not inconceivable that nicotine occupies binding sites that otherwise would be occupied by the paint solvents, with the result that the solvents cause less damage. One could say therefore that if you are painting indoors, you are better off smoking than not, at least with a view to the condition of your olfactory organ (we are not talking here about the harmful effects of smoking in general). Painting indoors is dangerous to the extent that these substances find their way to the brain relatively quickly (Chapter 2). Long-term exposure to substances like turpentine, cocaine and rubber solution has devastating effects on the nervous system. Nicotine can retard this process, insofar as the smoker does not die as the result of lung cancer or a heart attack.

Sex Differences

The olfactory capacity of women is superior to that of men on all fronts; on average the threshold value for many substances is considerably lower in women than in men,[140] and the whole hedonic palate of smells—the range of smell sensations—is wider and deeper in women. Women experience smells more intensely, and they are very clear as to whether they find a smell pleasant or unpleasant. Women also have a much more sensitive nose for body odors and are better able to distinguish men or women solely on the basis of the smell of sweat or breath.[141] Women also generally identify smells better than men do. As age increases, the differences between the sexes increase somewhat, because the olfactory capacity of men declines more quickly; put differently, the olfactory capacity of women in old age in absolute terms is less subject to decline. This fact accords with the general fact that women on average stay healthy and "intact" for longer than men.

Another difference is that women are better than men at giving names to smells. One reason for this: women generally have a better-developed language sense than men. This does not mean that women can always describe smells in detail: in both men and women there are only a limited number of direct connections between the rhinencephalon and the language centers, particularly in the neocortex. The cooperation between the two halves of the brain, it is supposed, is better in women than in men; this too might explain why women outscore men in giving names to smells.

In short, women perform better in all the known functions of smell. This is a general trend, independent of the culture to which one belongs, as has been shown by a research group at the University of Pennsylvania.[142] A smell test (UPSIT) was conducted with four groups of people: Japanese, black Americans, white Americans and Koreans who had lived in America for many

Smelling Scores

Group	Men	Women
Japanese	29.5	32.9
Blacks	32.4	34.0
Caucasians	33.6	34.2
Koreans	36.6	38.0

years.[143] In the various cultures, there are not inconsiderable differences among men and among women; within a population group, however, women always score better than men. Perhaps the discrepancies between the groups can be attributed partly to limitations in the method of research. One of the reasons for perceived differences may be that the odors used in the test were everyday and familiar in a Western society (perhaps affecting the Japanese differently than the whites). The group of whites also included more smokers. The Koreans had integrated into American society, and had a good nose for the smells used in this test. Note that the Korean man is even better at identifying smells than the average white woman, but this may be a result of the lower average age in the group of Koreans, which, moreover, included no smokers.

Another problem in this kind of experiment is that men and women, because of the customary division of labor, accumulate different experiences of smells. A man who seldom does the housekeeping will be less familiar with the smells of soap, vinegar and ammonia, whereas a housewife probably will have less to do with the smell of sawdust.

Let us consider another research project on the identifying capacity of men and women. The researchers presented the subjects with about eighty everyday smells, such as coffee, orange, vinegar, cigarette butts, banana, beer, chocolate, pepper, leather and cheese.[144] On average, the women were able to identify fifty of these smells correctly; the men approximately forty. Moreover, women showed more conviction or certainty, irrespective of whether they guessed correctly or wrongly. Men turned out to identify only fourteen of the eighty smells better than women (and then only slightly): mothballs, banana, peppermint, whiskey, sardines, ammonia, mustard, chewing gum, sawdust, black pepper, sherry, aftershave, syrup and raspberry lemonade. From these data it can be seen that the degree of familiarity with smells is not necessarily in itself decisive. That men should recognize the smell of aftershave better is not surprising, but what are we to make of their knack for recognizing ammonia or bananas? Moreover, the women were better at recognizing "masculine" smells such as pipe tobacco, rubber, machine oil and turpentine. One possible explanation for this is that many smells also act on the trigeminal nerve, which is supposed to be more sensitive in men than in women.

It is striking that the performance of both sexes improves considerably if the person conducting the experiment points out *incorrect* designations and corrects them. In an experiment on this point a list of smell names was prepared, and the subject had to name a presented odor from those on the list. Then the test subjects were asked to make such a list for themselves, which meant that they had to think of their own "label" whenever an odor was presented. In this case, too, the difference in performance between men and women remained. Even after about five sessions, when the subjects had to link the odors presented to them to the lists of names they had drawn up themselves, men performed the task less well than women. In a test consisting of forty odors, women were able to identify about 70 percent of smells correctly, men only 55 percent.

The sex differences at issue here emerge only in puberty; before that time boys and girls have approximately the same olfactory capacity. That during puberty girls' sense of smell starts getting better than that of boys is almost certainly due to the production of female sex hormones such as estrogen: if male rats are injected with estrogen, their sensitivity to smell improves. For the same reason women's sense of smell is keenest around the time of ovulation, when the concentration of estrogen is high.[145]

Another biological explanation for this might go as follows: Girls, from the point of view of natural selection, do not betray their ovulation to the outside world; because of this, during puberty they develop a nose for their own bodily odor, and, by extension, for all kinds of "domestic smells" (see Chapter 6). Boys, on the other hand (again reasoning from an evolutionary perspective), are more inclined during puberty to learn to reconnoiter a wide area around them; as a result, they are less interested in their bodily odors or in smells connected with the domestic sphere. Cultural evolution may have made up for these differences in development between girls and boys to some extent, but the biological mechanisms underlying them are still fully operational.

Smell and Culture

Research has also been carried out into the connections between one's olfactory capacity and the culture to which one belongs. In the case of the eye, we do not even consider such differences; there is no reason to assume that the eyes of a Chinese see any differently than ours (apart from aesthetic appreciation).[146] Smell is different. In the course of one's life the sense of smell is subject not only to great physiological differences but to anatomical ones as well. The number of sensory cells does not remain constant, nor does the ratio between the types of cells involved in smelling. Moreover, different societies are involved in different ways with substances that affect the olfactory organ, whether harmfully or beneficially.

This notion gains very little support from research, however. No essential differences in the olfactory capacity have been observed in people from different cultures (although it should be noted that test procedures are not always well adapted to the societies involved).[147] In fact, the sense of smell is quite similar from culture to culture. All people have approximately the same preferences regarding the smell of plants, spices, fruits and fresh water, and they all dislike the smell of rotting things and feces (except many young children). All over the world people prefer the body odors of their partner, children, family and friends to the body odors of strangers, which often cause a certain revulsion.[148]

The psychological and biological importance of this fairly rigid—or, to put it more favorably, fairly universal—appreciation of smells is obvious: man is looking for a suitable biotope, which explains the human preferences for certain plants and foods, as well as our dislike of rotting: likewise, in order to avoid infection it is sensible to avoid contact with feces.[149] And although man has not lived predominantly in small groups for a long time, he still likes a small-scale, highly structured environment full of recognizable and familiar smells.

There are marginal intercultural differences, of course. As is well known, the French like garlic more than the Dutch; Japanese find the smell of soap and perfume less pleasant than Germans and associate smells less with emotions than Germans do and more with personal hygiene. At the same time, Japanese make more explicit judgments on smells connected with their work, and respond less strongly to smells they come into contact with in their leisure time.[150]

Chapter 5

Smell and Memory

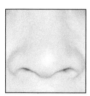An animal needs senses to investigate its environment for biological and social meanings and to adjust its behavior accordingly: elude predators, avoid dangerous or climatologically unfavorable circumstances, and seek opportunities for pleasure, if not by eating and drinking, then by finding a suitable candidate for cohabitation and/or reproduction. As far as smell is concerned, this principle is translated as follows: avoid stench and the dangerous objects connected with it, go in search of pleasant smells, and do not leave places that smell familiar, unless doing so is unavoidable.[151]

These behavioral mechanisms only operate, of course, when smell impressions are linked with experiences that are anchored in memory in some way. We shall concern ourselves with the question of how smell perceptions are stored, and consider in what way and to what extent memory traces, identifies, remembers, associates and describes smells.

Smell and Brain Activity

Smells seem to play a subsidiary role in human life; our perceptual existence would appear to be dominated by our eyes and ears. It has been estimated that 90 percent of all information that reaches us consciously does so through our capacity for sight. If smells (as it is claimed) are becoming less and less relevant in our lives, or if they begin to have negative effects on our chances of survival, then the consequences may be serious. The pressure of biological selection on the maintenance and development of our olfactory sense might so weaken that we would lose our capacity for smell.[152] After all, the mole is blind; for life underground, eyes are only a problem, because they can get dust and dirt in them.

However, the loss of the sense of smell, if it occurs, is unlikely to be rapid, despite Freud's assertion that our standing upright and walking account for the degeneration in our sense of smell. Smells influence our activity much more than we generally realize, and even affect our general level of brain activity (as has been measured with the EEG, the electroencephalogram). A few words about this.

It is remarkable that even breathing through the nose rather than through the mouth affects brain activity. Breathing through the nose not only increases the brain's sensitivity to smells—that is obvious—but the variation in the alpha and beta activity of the EEG (waves of 8-13 and 13-40 Hz, respectively) is greater when we breathe through the nose than when through the mouth.[153] This might mean that when we breathe through the nose, the brain is "more alert" and more ready to act. Smells also affect the activity of the right brain more than that of the left, as has been demonstrated with special scanning techniques.[154] This is an important fact, for the right hemisphere is relatively closely connected with emotions and with corresponding "crude motoric programs" such as taking flight.

What we smell while asleep, it turns out, affects our heartbeat and brain activity. Particularly during the first part of the night, the heartbeat quickens and EEG activity is increased if the smell of peppermint is administered now and again.[155] (These reactions also occur when other senses are stimulated: the electrical resistance of a sleeper's skin falls if his name is mentioned, which points to a certain activation based on subconscious information processing.) In addition to smells that increase wakefulness, there may be fragrances that have an opposite effect, improving sleep. And it has been shown that fragrances presented in low concentrations—so low that they cannot be perceived consciously—sometimes also lead to considerably diverging EEG patterns. No explanation has been found for this; it might mean that our conscious perception of a smell does not say everything about its meaning for us.[156]

It has even been shown that smells that test subjects experience consciously and (in intensity and quality) regard as virtually identical sometimes are linked with very different brain-wave patterns. That phenomenon, too, is as yet not understood; it is obviously possible that a conscious experience is an unreliable or at least an incomplete indication of the "actual" impression that the smell makes on the brain as a whole. A conceivable consequence of this phenomenon is that a smell's effect on behavior does not completely accord with our conscious experience and appreciation of it. This point requires a rather technical explanation, which, moreover, does not completely explain the phenomena that have just been described.

In every smell perception the olfactory bulbus as a whole is involved.[157] When a smell is inhaled, the bulbus becomes more sensitive and increases its electrical activity. Through positive feedback in the system (signals are reinforced rather than weakened), at a certain moment such a degree of instability is created that the bulbus fires a pattern of signals (a "burst"). Such a pattern or burst varies from smell to smell and forms the neurophysiological basis of the process of identifying and distinguishing smells. In exhalation, the stimulus declines, the sensitivity of the bulbus reduces greatly, and the signal weakens. The important point now is that the condition and operation of the system as a whole is determined both by the properties of the smells inhaled and by various other processes, which take place at the same moment in the central nervous system.[158]

This means, among other things, that through the making of associations a smell may after a passage of time display a completely different signal pattern than previously. For example, sawdust evokes a specific pattern in the electrical activity of the bulbus. If a mixture of the smell of banana and sawdust is presented a number of times, and then only the smell of sawdust, it turns out that the original (sawdust) pattern is considerably changed for a certain period of time. It looks therefore as though the operation of the bulbus is constantly changing; and those changes help to determine the characteristics of the final signal. Put simply: what you smell also depends on what you have (just) smelled. The olfactory sensation is not a perception which is created *linea recta* (which, moreover, is not the case with any sense); what we smell is partly also determined by recent history.

As has been said, odors turn out to be capable of affecting processes on various levels in the central nervous system. The reverse is also true: the general condition of the brain affects the processing and experience of smells. There is no one-way traffic. More generally, we can state that our capacity for smell is greatly affected by our overall physical and physiological condition. This form of flexibility or sensitivity of the olfactory system manifests itself as enormous differences in sensitivity and appreciation of smells in the same person (*alliesthesia*). This kind of feedback to a sense from the brain and the body is unusual, for it is lacking in hearing and sight.[159]

Neurophysiological Imprinting of Smells

Rats are also used frequently in research in the field of olfactory memory, for they have an excellent sense of smell (they are macrosmates) and have a good memory for smells.

Where is the memory for smell located in the brain? Researchers undertook the following experiment in an attempt to answer this question.

Young rats were conditioned by stimulating one of the two olfactory organs ten times with the smell of cedar. This was carried out through one nostril; the other was blocked with a plug. At the same time the animals were fed milk through a tube.[160] Subsequently the stimulated nostril was closed and the other opened. Half an hour later the rats were given a choice between two habitats: a cage with the smell of cedar and one without. The rats turned out to spend more time in the cage with the smell of cedar. Obviously this smell was associated via conditioning with milk, for the animal a pleasant association. This finding is remarkable, since the links between the sense of smell and the brain do not cross. Since the information stored in one half of the brain during the conditioning process turned out to be accessible to the opposite olfactory organ, we have to assume that smell centers in the brain communicate via a crossed link (Chapter 3).[161] Very young rats cannot be conditioned in this way: the creatures must be over twelve days old, because the connections between the two halves of the brain have to mature before exchange of information between the hemispheres is possible. That phenomenon is also familiar in man: the cooperation between our hemispheres reaches optimum efficiency only after about eight years.

As soon as the cross-connections are functioning properly, previous experiences turn out to be accessible to the other olfactory organ. If rats six days old are conditioned in the way described above and are tested only six days later with the other nostril open, they also show a preference for the cage with the smell of cedar. This preference, however, does not exist in rats between six and twelve days old during the second test. Conclusion: the cross-connections relevant to smell function well in rats after twelve days; from that moment on, earlier experiences become accessible to the other hemisphere. The connection concerned—the *commissura anterior*—is the foremost of the three most important links between the hemispheres.

The next question: is all information stored on both sides once the links are mature and operational? That is: does the right hemisphere receive a "copy" of the information which the left-hand olfactory organ has passed on to the left hemisphere? An experiment shows that this is not the case. If in older rats one first severs the foremost cross-connection between the hemispheres after a conditioning experiment such as the one described above, the animals still prefer the cage with the smell of cedar, provided they smell via the trained olfactory organ. If that nostril is blocked and the animals therefore are able to smell only through the other nostril, the preference disappears. In short: in the field of smell there is communication between the hemispheres but they are not by definition double-storage (none of this applies if both nostrils are used, but that is obvious). Since the nostrils both in man and in rats are equally accessible (think of the nasal rhythm), this form of communication is of great importance. The cross-connections ensure that the storage capacity of the rhinencephalon is used efficiently: if information is transported from the left-hand olfactory organ to the left side of the brain, the latter is also accessible to the right hemisphere. The sense of smell in rats, therefore, operates in a far from rigid way. This is a quite unusual finding, for systems that appeared long ago in evolution are frequently fairly rectilinear or rigid.[162]

Remarkable observations about man have also been made in this field. In the 1950s, the largest cross-connection between the hemispheres (the *corpus callosum*) was severed in a number of patients to combat serious forms of epilepsy. From that moment on, these people were no longer or scarcely able to give names to smells administered via the right-hand nostril, but they were occasionally able to identify those presented through the left nostril.[163] This finding tallies with the animal experiments we just mentioned and with the fact that the left hemisphere is much more connected with language than its right-hand neighbor. Continuing this reasoning, one might suspect that the *quality* of a smell would also depend somewhat on the combination of nostril-hemisphere, because the right hemisphere is slightly more involved in emotions and feelings than the left one.[164] No specific research has been conducted into this question, however.

A second observation indicates that patients in whom the right-hand temporal lobe of the cortex has been damaged can no longer say whether smells are connected with one another. In this regard, think of the link that we make between the smell of a burning candle and that of the wick that has just been extinguished; we are aware that there is a connection between the smell of tobacco and the smell of a half-finished cigarette; we recognize a relationship between the smell of butter and that of gravy. These people, however, are no longer able to do this. Their capacity to perceive smells separately has not been affected, but they can no longer make certain connections.[165] Pathological processes therefore show that the center of gravity of the processing of smell impressions is situated in the right hemisphere.[166] The fact that the right hemisphere makes all kinds of connections between olfactory stimuli we perceive also applies to other senses. For example, the perception of complex patterns such as faces is mainly a task of this hemisphere. A trivial injury to a small area in this half of the brain can produce *prosopagnosia*, the inability to recognize faces.

We repeat: the rat has a well-developed olfactory memory.[167] It can easily be conditioned to approximately thirty smells, with more than five attempts at conditioning per smell rarely being necessary. Even if one waits a month after the learning phase before conducting a smell test, the rat does not perform any worse than immediately afterward. In addition, rats retain smells given a negative significance (for example, by the application of an electric shock) just as well as they do smells with a positive one (for example, the combination of the smell of cedar and milk). The rat can experience *and* retain a smell either as an alarm signal or as a pleasant stimulus. The same applies to humans: children retain a smell linked to a pleasant photograph just as well as an odor accompanied by a photograph that they don't like.[168] Gradually, however, a shift takes place in the appreciation of smell; odors linked to appealing photographs begin to smell more pleasant, at least in six-year-olds, a phenomenon that can be understood on the basis of the laws of conditioning. In ten-year-olds, the experience of smell and the appreciation of smell have become much more stable. Slightly older children know more qualities of smells, which means that a conditioning experiment cannot change them so easily. Moreover, children at that age can think more logically than six-year-olds, and so behave more critically in smell tests.

A smell, once imprinted in the memory, is also recognized by the rat in a not too complicated mixture of smells. Humans, however, are beginners in this field: we perform rather badly in analyzing mixtures. It is not known what the basis of this difference is. Our smell memory is like a system in which stimuli are stored as a whole ("gestalt"), like names, gestures, faces, shapes, "our front door" and suchlike. Such a memory system does not focus so much on details, but records mainly the overall picture. This explanation is not satisfactory, however. Often we can recognize other people by seeing only one part of their face, read a sentence reasonably well even if some of the letters (or even parts of all the letters) are missing, decipher a neon sign, with two tubes out of order, reading *Phlps.* The analogy, then, does not apply; onc would expect that with a kind of smell memory comparable to our capacity for sight, we would be able to recognize a smell *fragment* in a mixture, but that is precisely what we are not very good at.

Retention of Smells

The memory of human beings and animals is classified in different ways. There is a short-term and a long-term memory; an explicit memory and an implicit memory (which influences our behavior through experiences of which we are not aware, such as events that take place during sleep or while we are under anesthetic); a retrospective or cpisodic memory (for events that have taken place and that we also know about); and a prospective memory, which makes it possible for us to perform what we were intending to do a quarter of an hour ago.

The distinction between the *episodic* and the *semantic* memory is very important. With the episodic memory, we are able to remember many events, including a large part of our life history. With the semantic memory, we can recognize phenomena and objects and describe them in language. Where a car came from and how fast it was going are episodic facts; your being able to identify an object coming toward you as fast as a car is a semantic fact.

Both these types of memory processes are involved in smell. When we smell something, we attach a great deal of meaning to the emotional, hedonic and episodic associations of the smell. Episodic connections particularly are evoked by smells; meanings at the semantic level play a less pregnant part in smell, because we are either unable or scarcely able to describe many smells. At the level of language we are often not even able to place a fragrance. By way of analogy, think of the traffic again: something rushes past, but you don't know whether it is a moped or a light motorcycle. Despite the presence of lucid olfactory impressions we are unable to identify the source or substance of the smell precisely, which means that our capacity to trace smells back to the semantic domain is very limited.[169] To be quite clear: someone who *sees* a banana recognizes the smell effortlessly, but if a piece of banana is put into a jar under a wad of cotton wool, there is a good chance that he or she will have trouble identifying it.

One aspect of this phenomenon has already been mentioned: smells mainly stimulate the limbic system and the right hemisphere, neither of which has much to do with our linguistic capacities. (It is possible to make a case as to why women are slightly better able to describe smells than men: there are indications that the hemispheres in women communicate rather more intensively than in men, partly because the cross-connections between the hemispheres are generally better developed in women.)

From a neurophysiological and psychological point of view, the identification of smells is a complicated process, one that takes a relatively large amount of time—as a rule, a few seconds.[170] The smell has to be decoded, and that happens in an inefficient and sometimes arbitrary manner, certainly when we take the speed and effectiveness of other senses into account. Potential labels or meanings have to be activated from the semantic memory, a process that occurs slowly and produces inconsistent results. Next a label has to be selected, and there can be competition between various designations: the smell of old cheese can also be that of sweaty feet. It generally does not take much effort to establish that something stinks or smells pleasant, but expressing *precisely* what "stinking" or "smelling pleasant" means causes problems. Sometimes naming is not successful even with familiar smells; generally the other senses are needed in order to trace a smell impression back to a precise source, cause and name, as can be seen from the example of the banana. That is not unusual, though. The naming and placing of smells do not play important parts in everyday life: our capacity to distinguish dangerous and harmless smells is reasonably well developed, and that is what matters most.

In evolutionary terms, this is all perfectly understandable: the precise identification of smells has only limited use. We perceive a smell, and its positive or negative *signal* is communicated; just what substance we are smelling is of secondary importance. One can think in this connection of emotions, which are general programs that shape our behavior. Emotions are directed at satisfying our elementary needs.[171] Because emotions serve our interests in a general sense, perceived stimuli at the level of behavior are divided into about four classes only: "continue," "stop," "good," "bad." Because smells are closely bound up with emotions, a "coarse" (that is, a scarcely semantic) processing of the information is sufficient to promote these general interests.

How does smell function in people who have one or more of their senses missing? Blind people are better at identifying smells than sighted people.[172] The difference is quite great indeed: blind people are able to name many more smells correctly, even though for unknown reasons they are less able to recognize a number of specific smells, such as those of liverwurst, cigar butts, toast, popcorn and mothballs. Blind people can recognize and name honey, cloves, bleach, onions, coffee and banana better and quicker than sighted people. The reason for this is obvious: blind people have relatively more difficulty in localizing the source of a smell, which means that they have to focus more on the properties of the smell itself. It does not follow from this that blind people have a *more sensitive* olfactory organ. On the contrary: the threshold value for detection of many odors is substantially higher for them. So the commonly held belief that because of their handicap blind people are able to smell (and hear and feel) better must be qualified. Particularly if blindness (in children) is a result of a severe illness such as meningitis, or an ailment affecting the whole body —such as a venereal disease transmitted by the mother during pregnancy—then other senses may not develop properly either.

The inability to name smells can be improved somewhat; even

people with excellent vision are capable in principle of learning and using a reference system for smells. Perfumers and other smell professionals are often very proud of this, although their performance should not be overestimated.[173] Nevertheless, it would be useful if we were able to identify smells somewhat better. Fortunately, the eye and the ear also help language a little. For example, androsterone, a male pheromone, is detected more easily if a name is given to the smell.[174] The basis for this may be that perception, with the help of language, can be sharpened somewhat, a mechanism called the *Sapir-Whorf hypothesis*: when you have a word for something, the object in question can sometimes be more easily distinguished from other things. For example, many people tend to say that brick walls can be laid in only one way (the stretcher bond), but a tour of the town with a bricklayer will lead them to see many more kinds of walls (random bond, Flemish bond, etc.).

The same principle has emerged from research into how we distinguish subtle differences in color. If one works with people who cannot perceive any difference between certain tints and presents them many times with the same colors *and* designations, their ability to distinguish colors appears to improve somewhat. Analogously, various experiments have shown that the names and descriptions of smells can help a person to detect and recognize smells.[175] The "twofold coding theory" provides an explanation for this. A person retains information better if it is established (coded) doubly—semantically (one word, one code) *and* in the "language" of a sensory system itself. In other words, it is more difficult to remember just a smell than a smell that has an appropriate label or meaning; in the latter case, you have two "hooks" available. To take another example, retaining a portion of straight text turns out to be more difficult than recalling a text that during the learning phase was accompanied by illustrations; in this case, too, double coding plays a part.

As far as smell is concerned, however, the research data are not so reliable and unambiguous.[176] You can imagine that the test subjects in such experiments would not remember the smells, but rather their labels or meanings. As a rule, we do our best to score well in a memory test; for that reason it is conceivable that the contribution of the verbal memory masks that of the actual smell memory. Moreover, one can (consciously or unconsciously) cheat through logical reflection and verbalization—that is, someone has retained the smell labels without properly recognizing the accompanying smells as such: "This smell is probably not A, so probably it was B that was meant, although I can't recognize it now." Think again, by way of (a rather poor) analogy, of how we retain the content of books versus how we remember a list of titles. The situation can be compared somewhat with a multiple-choice test. For example: pi is a number. Give the value of pi:

a. Jan is ill.
b. Peter has a bike.
c. 3.14.
d. Friday.

The answer is definitely not a, b or d, so c is the right answer. Because you understand language you can find the right answer without knowing anything about pi.

The implicit memory also plays a part in the sense of smell. It concerns things that we store unintentionally, unconsciously or without effort and retain, and that we are not even *aware* of knowing, but that nevertheless influence our behavior. Even during a general anesthetic we absorb information through hearing, such as the surgeon's comments in the operating room. This information finds its way into the implicit memory. Next, our mood and rate of recovery are affected by such (less pleasant) pronouncements, though we have no memory of them. In gallbladder operations, putting headphones on the patient so that it is *impossible* for her to hear what is being said about her condition during the operation shortens the period of hospitalization by no less than 15 or 20 percent. (With the appropriate positive suggestions one can achieve even more, but this simple money-saving method is scarcely ever used.[177]) Even in a state of deep unconsciousness, the implicit memory still works to a certain extent. In one instance, a patient who had been lying in a coma for a long time was washed with jasmine soap, a type of soap that he did not know. When he recovered consciousness, he recognized the smell of the soap.

In amnesia patients, mainly the explicit memory is affected. These people find it difficult to repeat words from a list that they have been given a short while before. If you ask them to associate freely on an arbitrarily chosen word, then they give almost as many words from the list as people who don't have any problem with memory. We can conclude from this that the implicit memory is affected less than the explicit memory. Research in the field of smell memory, unfortunately, rarely takes account of this intriguing process and difference.

Another question: does a previous confrontation with a different smell have a positive effect on one's naming of a smell? An example: when you smell sprouts for the first time, can you subsequently place the smell of a mincemeat ball better? Does the smell of oregano help you to identify spaghetti sauce? The recognition of a certain kind of substance can indeed make the detection of a related substance easier; that is probably because the semantic frame of reference in this case helps one a little. Whatever the case, opinions are divided on the question of how precisely the smell memory works. There is a group of researchers who believe that this memory is not basically different from visual memory.[178] Others disagree; they maintain that smell perceptions are scarcely ever decoded in the abstract and that (therefore) they are stored as unique, crude and also scarcely interchangeable impressions.[179] One can understand this view: smell impressions are not directly connected with abstracting systems in our brain (recall that smell, in evolutionary terms, is an old sense), and the meaning of a smell is in the first place hedonic and non-cognitive in nature. As has been observed, this also emerges from recording the electrical activity in the brain: the right hemisphere is dominant in the recognition of smells, while the comprehension and use of language are mainly jobs for the left hemisphere.

Evolutionary arguments can be adduced to explain this general division of labor, which was discussed in part previously. The right hemisphere contains mainly motor programs of a crude or general nature, connected with emotional reactions (such as running away); the left hemisphere contains mainly programs for refined motor functions and language. Because smells are principally connected with emotions, and because they also often have an alarm function, it is obvious that such a signal should be linked to crude motor function programs.[180] Again and briefly, an important function of smell seems to be that of linking concrete behavioral reactions to concrete olfactory sensations; cognitive and intellectual aims or functions are not paramount.[181] For example, people find it difficult to "imagine" or "evoke" smells, in the way that you can call up the Eiffel Tower in your mind's eye. Some 40 percent of people maintain that they are able to do this.[182] However, the identification of smells does not improve if the test subject is asked to do his best to imagine the smells as well.[183] According to other experiments, only a few people are able to do this to any extent.

Consider this odd phenomenon connected with the smell memory.[184] Suppose you have someone smell an odor and then ask the person to let you know when they perceive that smell again. If you present the same smell three seconds later, a smaller percentage of test subjects recognize the smell than when you wait for twelve seconds. That is fairly logical, one may say—an effective adaptation. Things are not that simple, however. If you wait still longer, then the percentage of people scoring correctly falls, and at about thirty seconds you have the same result as in the three-second test. The recognition *peak* is around twelve seconds. Why is that? With images and sounds there is no possibility of such a late optimum point. Compared with other senses, the smell memory requires a lot of time to store the information. Moreover, this process proceeds in a far from thoughtless way. The number of incorrect pronouncements is relatively large: approximately 20 percent of test subjects say that they recognize the smell at moments when it is not even present ("false alarm"). Apart from that, the intensity of the smell to be retained is always assessed at a lower level than in reality, which may be a consolation to people with chronically sweaty feet or very smelly armpits.[185]

The recognition of a smell also declines if you have the test subject smell a second smell shortly after the first is presented.[186]

It is assumed that the new smell impression interferes with the storage of the first smell and that in this way "ready knowledge" is affected. If you do not cause a subject to smell a second smell in the meantime, but ask the subject to perform another task (such as counting backward), then this effect scarcely occurs. Nor does repeating the name of the presented smell cause any disruption; giving a name helps in recognition. We observed that in a different context: the smell impression is now also coded and retained via language. The name, rather than interfering, helps the smell memory in identification. This is also shown by the following: if you have the test subject repeat the name of a different smell, that makes almost no difference to the recognition of the smell concerned.

If short-term recognition of smells is sometimes faulty, certainly compared with the recognition of images and sounds, the long-term smell memory functions much better. What has once—albeit with the necessary difficulty—been etched in the olfactory memory is stored for a considerable time. It has been shown by many experiments that smells remembered after a day are generally still remembered a month later, and even after a year the smell memory still performs reasonably well.[187] (In this respect, too, the smell memory of women operates slightly better than that of men.)

One common but debatable view of smell memory maintains (as we saw previously) that a smell sensation is retained as an overall impression ("gestalt"), so that the mechanism is supposed to suffer little disturbance from other perceptions. However, that is not completely true: when another smell is presented, the recognition process does proceed less effectively. That phenomenon applies to other senses as well. A visual stimulus (such as an illustration from a holiday brochure) is eventually forgotten, partly and particularly because so many different elements have to be retained. Other perceptions also can disturb the memory of the original illustration. Less detailed or very familiar illustrations therefore are retained better in the long term than are complex or unknown pictures. The same principle seems to apply to smell: the more complicated or unfamiliar smells (mixtures) are, the more inefficiently they are retained.[188] But whether this means that there is no fundamental difference between the visual memory and the olfactory memory is not known.

Smells as Memory Aids

Many people will recognize the sweet smell of oatmeal even though they have not eaten the stuff for years. And the smell of the cakes which brightened the breaks at nursery school is fixed indelibly in many people's memories. Even if one does not experience the smell again for forty years, one still may recognize it in a smell test. That is a remarkable fact, since after so many years one cannot recall other essential things from that time, such as the name or even the appearance of the teacher or the number of children in the class. If one sniffs the cake for a longer time, then often other memories from that time emerge; if someone is scarcely able to say anything about his years in elementary school, the smell of chalk can help him to remember certain things. In other words, smells activate the episodic memory. Sometimes the sense of smell can function as a kind of "starter motor" that evokes all kinds of apparently forgotten experiences and events from the past, even though sometimes one cannot name or describe the smell concerned more precisely.

This mechanism is called *state-dependent retrieval.* What a person has learned in a particular physiological state, a certain mental state or in a certain place, she later can remember perfectly well under the same circumstances. Examples: if someone learns a list of words by heart in a state of slight intoxication, they'll reproduce it better if they have a drink first; a diver performs worse in listing words on the surface than he was able to do in the learning phase underwater.[189] From this it follows that eyewitnesses of accidents or crimes perform better when they tell their story to the police where the scene actually happened; the surroundings activate their memories.[190]

This form of conditioning also functions in regard to one's mood. In one experiment, test subjects were asked to keep a diary for a number of months. At a certain point they were asked to write a summary. Those who felt gloomy at that time wrote down a relatively sad story, but those who felt cheerful focused on pleasant events. When the stories were checked against the complete diaries, it emerged that the differences between stories and diaries were not based on "lying," but on a process of unconscious selection. If you are depressed, you feel that your life is a succession of sad scenes. An infamous artifact in this context is the notion that cancer patients have often had "unhappy childhoods." Often that is not the case: these people's memories are colored by the gloomy mood induced by the diagnosis.[191]

But back to our starting point: smells can also serve as memory aids, and a smell can evoke a certain mood with the attendant memories. Often the memory images that emerge through smells have a decidedly emotional charge, due to the connections between the sense of smell and the limbic system and the right hemisphere of the brain.[192] In an experiment, test subjects were asked what memories were evoked by twenty everyday smells, varying from peppermint to sweaty socks. In many cases a smell did lead the subject to a memory picture, although the person often could not place the smell very well. For a large percentage of the test subjects, the memories were very vivid and emotionally colored. Almost two-thirds of the images were connected with events from at least a year previously, and more than a quarter related to childhood (possibly because the test subjects were students of about twenty). Differences were found between men and women. The terminology used by women was generally more emotional in nature, and their memories were slightly clearer or more vivid than those of the men.

It also emerged that one remembers more pleasant things when in pleasant-smelling surroundings. In other words, smelling a pleasant smell goes hand in hand with recalling pleasant memories.[193] This link pulls two ways, though, and it does not function the same way with everyone. Of course, not all kinds of smells are inherently or "necessarily" pleasant. The point is that a pleasant experience connected with a particular smell perception *makes* that smell pleasant in nature through conditioning. Alternatively, someone is put into a pleasant mood by the smell in question, which ensures that mainly pleasant memories emerge.

The reverse is also true: think of the unpleasant associations that arise when you smell the typical smell of a hospital. In theory, hospitals would be well advised to replace their characteristic smell through air conditioning, not least because negative ideas and gloominess in patients lead to a slower recovery.

The link between smells and memory is more than a link between the present and the past; one can also use it in learning various things. A list of words learned by heart will be reproduced better in an area perfumed with jasmine if one first learned the words in a jasmine-scented room; the smell activates the semantic memory for the words concerned.[194] The same applies to the recognition of people from passport photographs.[195] Jasmine does not have a monopoly on this: in such experiments it makes little difference whether the room smells nice or stinks; in principle, any smell can act as a memory aid via conditioning. Neutral or unknown smells that do not yet evoke any emotions, are, however, the most effective, since they can be linked with a new situation relatively easily. (Thiol, however, is so strongly associated with natural gas that that smell is less than suitable for this kind of experiment.)

In short, smells can serve as memory aids or as means of conditioning reactions and performance; a smell that is neutral in itself can be given a meaning through association with the context within which it is perceived. Through this form of conditioning it is possible to link mood and performance to each other, as the following indicates.[196] A number of people were asked to copy complicated patterns with the aid of blocks, as part of an intelligence test (the WAIS: Wechsler Adult Intelligence Scale). In half of the cases, the instruction sheet used for the test was impregnated with a substance called trimethylundecylenic aldehyde (TUA), a neutral odor that evokes no specific associations or feelings. In a second session subjects were asked to judge photographs of men and women on the basis of a questionnaire. They were asked to describe the "emotional" impression the photographed people made on them: tense-relaxed, worried-content, nervous-calm, unfriendly-friendly, attractive-unattractive. The following emerged from the results. The female test subjects, particularly, who had had great difficulty in making the patterns, judged the photos much more negatively when they smelled the TUA smell from the first session.[197] That is, the stress they had felt in solving the puzzle was "generalized" to another task. A second questionnaire, which assessed the mood of the test subjects, showed that the TUA group felt more anxious during the second session than the control group. This phenomenon, a form of fear of failure, occurred more in the female test subjects than in the males. This did not apply to the test subjects who had also had problems in solving the block patterns but who in the first instance had been given an odorless instruction sheet.

The group was small—twelve men and twelve women—so one cannot conclude that women can be more easily conditioned to smells than men. Even so, this experiment makes clear that smell, linked to the execution of tasks, can evoke emotions or moods or reinforce them. A smell, neutral in itself, was linked to the "stress" brought on by a difficult task; merely the exposure to that smell appears capable of reawakening the feeling of stress or fear. This kind of conditioning occurs at an unconscious level; when the test subjects were asked after the conclusion of the experiment whether they had any idea of the aim of the research and whether they had noticed anything special, none was able to link the two sessions. As a verification, the odor was presented again, and the subjects were asked if they had smelled it before. Only one-sixth recognized it, and only two people remembered noticing it during the experiment. Such phenomena have been observed outside the laboratory as well. An example from daily life: A woman was caught in an elevator for two hours because of a power failure. She was wearing perfume at the time, and when she used it again she had an attack of claustrophobia; naturally she lost the desire to buy the scent again.[198]

The experiment and the example above point (yet again) to the important signaling function of smells. When you are put under pressure because you have to carry out a complicated task and there is a specific smell in the surroundings, then that smell, when present while you are engaged in a new task, acts as a sign to anticipate effort. That "feeling of stress" presents itself even when there is no need to get tense, as in the instance above in which the photographs were judged. Smells can make us act and feel in a certain way via a learning process.

On the basis of this it will also be clear that smells do not *by definition* have a positive or negative influence on performance during an examination or anything else; they involve mainly associations and learning processes, including simple conditioning. Yet it is conceivable that a student will do better on an exam if there is the same smell in the examination room as there was at home, where he was studying.

Only occasionally does smell directly affect the capacity to learn. For example, lavender helps a person perform mathematical calculations faster and with fewer errors. Lavender has a relaxing effect, which is not consonant with the (active) attitude expected in mathematics.[199] But lavender might have an especially favorable effect on a student with both a flair for mathematics and a fear of examinations (lavender is sometimes called "student's herb").

There are several examples in contemporary life. At London's Heathrow Airport, the scent of pine needles is sprayed in the terminals: in this way an attempt is made to put people at their ease (taking no account of those patrons who got lost in the forest in their youth and who have associated the smell of pine needles with fear ever since). Because the smell of lemon appears to help clerical workers to make fewer mistakes in entering data in computers and in word processing, some companies now disseminate the smell of lemon via the air conditioning. In many Japanese companies it is even customary to add different smells to the air in the course of the day: a little lemon in the mornings, then a light flowery smell and during the afternoon (to keep up morale) the smell of wood.[200] Smells are used to keep customers in shops. In department stores it appears that more running shoes are sold if there is a smell of flowers in the shoe department, and old cars are more attractive if they are given the smell of new cars with a spray can. In the United States, some entrepreneurs have marketed spray cans with the smell of clean rooms. And it has been proposed that one way to protect telephone booths against vandalism would be to treat them with aggression-calming fragrances (such as baby oil). It might even be possible to equip football stadiums with enormous smell disseminators, which would kick in and release mellowing fragrances at the first threat of a fight between fans.[201]

Again, we must realize that the link between smells and sales is a loose one: there is no evidence that smells stimulate the *general* desire to purchase. It is, however, possible to use existing associations. A motorist who has a vague desire for a cup of coffee as he pulls into a gas station during a long drive may be convinced to have a cup by the smell of fresh coffee brewing in the attendant's office; someone who is toying with the idea of buying a Christmas tree may be more inclined actually to buy because of the smell of the tree. However, these associations are completely different from the widespread misunderstanding that the "smell columns" in department stores—which spread all kinds of pleasant smells—cause people to buy diverse products: nothing of the kind has been shown.

The fact that smells can have certain effects on behavior has in a certain sense been known for a long time. "Let the rest rooms and bedrooms, the studies, the dining rooms and bathrooms be surrounded by pleasant smells," an expert in the field of garden design wrote in 1771. "The pleasure of these perfumes brings an indescribable relaxation and peace to man's heart, filling it with a warm feeling of satisfaction."[202]

The Link with Colors

Smell is a strange sense. Our nose is able to distinguish a large percentage of the estimated 400,000 known odors, but if you ask someone to put a name to a smell, then he or she is often dumbstruck.[203] A smell (in a bottle) is found to be pleasant or unpleasant; in a number of cases we manage to identify the possible source or nature of the substance, but normally a correct diagnosis is not given. If the eye were to function like the nose, when you saw a sheet of bright red paper you would say something like "Looks furious" rather than "Sheet of red paper." The related Bordeaux red would evoke a completely different reaction, such as

"Makes a warm impression" or "Looks very tasty, is something like wine." The reverse is also true: physically totally different stimuli, for example a bilious green object and a bright red one, might be judged almost identical if the eye were to see the way the nose smells—namely, primarily sensitive to and focused on the hedonic quality and the emotional charge of the stimulus.

There is an intriguing interaction between smells and colors. It has been shown that the perceived intensity of a smell increases if the odorant (in a bottle) is given a color.[204] This phenomenon also occurs if one adds unusual and non-matching colors: red to the smell of lemons, green to the smell of strawberries. In this experiment the test subjects are generally not aware that there is such an interaction between smells and colors, and they are surprised to learn that the colorless mixture of smell is just as strong as the colored one. Some refuse to believe this, maintaining that the researchers have made a mistake. This can be called an example of "perceptual anticipation" of the olfactory impression evoked by a color. We may reason in our unconscious that things that are colorless will also be odorless and tasteless; moreover, it may be that senses have a directly reinforcing effect on each other. This latter is called "intermodal interaction."

Another cause of the connections between colors and smells is that things that smell pleasant or unpleasant generally have an "accompanying" beautiful or ugly color. Some colors are even so strongly associated with certain smells that the application of another color falsifies the smell impression. If a cherry drink is colored yellowy orange, people often find that the liquid smells of orange, taking it to be orange juice or something similar. Fruit juice often consists of a mixture of different fruit extracts; the smell and taste experience is driven mainly by the color of the drink: cassis is black, tomato juice red. An unanswered question is why perfume is almost always yellow or the color of urine. Probably it is simply the intention that the substance should not be visible on the skin.

These kinds of links between smells and colors can also arise via conditioning or as a result of previous experiences. Perhaps experiences of all kinds lead the nervous system to make synaptic links between the systems that encode smells and colors. This is not very probable, though; after all, the rhinencephalon is a long way from the visual system. Yet we cannot exclude the possibility that even from birth there are neural connections between the visual and olfactory systems. An indication in the direction might be the following.

Initially babies are scarcely able to separate the information from their various sensory systems. Very young children mix all impressions together. That phenomenon is called *synesthesia*; in older children and adults a light stimulus may be strongly associated with a particular sound, or when one listens to music one also sees colors. In a small number of cases this early-childhood confusion continues into the person's later life; such people have difficulty in distinguishing images from sounds. All sensory information is "put together" or mixed. In order to perceive an image as an image, a smell as a smell and a sound as a sound, a splitting of systems or "modules" is necessary at the anatomical level, too. Possibly a remnant of the original "diffuse network" continues to exist, which would help to explain the influence of colors on the perception of smells.[205] To put it differently, synesthesia in the young child is based on a "crude" form of information processing. The neocortex of the newborn child lacks the microstructure necessary for it to operate efficiently. Partly as a result, in the child's world of experience everything seems connected with everything else; only later are separate channels opened in the cortex for each sense. This process, however, does not always lead to a complete division of systems.

The fact that synesthesia does have an anatomical background emerges from the following observation in people who associate sounds with colors. The argument is that blood from language systems in the left cortex flows to areas connected with seeing colors. In a certain sense, then, there is a "barrier" missing, allowing the two to be linked.[206]

Language and Literature

Again, our terminology for describing smells is generally meager or inadequate, due to our neural architecture. The parts of the brain that are closely involved in the use of language have few direct links with the olfactory system. Because consciousness and the use of language are closely connected, it is understandable why olfactory information plays a part mainly on an unconscious level.

However, there are still some unanswered questions relating to this inadequate and limited terminology. Is the phenomenon connected mainly with smells themselves, which are indeed difficult to divide into classes (Chapter 3), or is it a kind of incapacity that can be traced back to the construction of our brains? Is the meaning of what you smell, for example, comparable with the physical expression of rage and aggression, a process which is under the control of the unconsciously operating brain stem or the "neural chassis" and which is not generally associated with careful and grammatically correct language usage? It is difficult to say anything sensible about this subject: relatively little is known about the precise way in which various sections of the brain work and communicate with each other.

If we want to determine and name the quality of a smell, we often use terms derived from other sensory systems. Many words for smells belong as well to taste (sour, sweet, rancid, bitter, sharp, fine, tasty, revolting), to touch (warm, cool, heavy, fresh), to hearing (harmonious, melodious) or to sight (clear, vague, dark). Adjectives directly connected to the perception of a smell are generally derived from the associated nouns (odor, stink, smell, whiff). There aren't very many such words: stuffy, overwhelming, stinking, rotting, penetrating, pungent, fragrant, perfumed, volatile . . . Does our limited verbal expressiveness in this area have a purely biological or neurophysiological background or is there more involved? Perhaps the reason is that smells are not regarded as very important in modern cultures, and perhaps there was even a period when language was "deodorized" (Chapter 1). Language usage relating to smells may have *become* rather impoverished. In the same way, the language of smell could become richer and more varied if smells were given greater prestige.[207]

The Dutch expression "to tell something in smells and colors" means to give a vivid account, but do we actually do that? Colors occur frequently in novels and stories, smell much less often. We are usually satisfied with statements like "This smells like coffee," and "This smell is a little like orange." In the well-known olfactory novel *Perfume*, by Patrick Süskind, this method—that is, referring to an object to describe or designate a smell—is used relentlessly, as in this excerpt:

"In the period of which we speak, there reigned in the cities a stench barely conceivable to us modern men and women. The streets stank of manure, the courtyards of urine. The stairwells stank of moldering wood and rat droppings, the kitchens of spoiled cabbage and mutton fat; the unaired parlors stank of stale dust, the bedrooms of greasy sheets, damp feather beds and the pungently sweet aroma of chamber pots. The stench of sulphur rose from the chimneys, the stench of caustic lyes from the tanneries, and from the slaughterhouses came the stench of congealed blood. People stank of sweat and unwashed clothes; from their mouths came the stench of rotting teeth, from their bellies that of onions, and from their bodies, if they were no longer very young, came the stench of rancid cheese and sour milk and tumorous disease. The rivers stank, the marketplaces stank, the churches stank, it stank beneath the bridges and in the palaces. The peasant stank, as did the priest, the apprentice as did his master's wife, the whole of the aristocracy stank, even the King himself stank, stank like a rank lion, and the Queen like an old goat, summer and winter. For in the eighteenth century there was nothing to hinder bacteria busy at decomposition, and so there was no human activity either constructive or destructive, no manifestation of germinating or decaying life, that was not accompanied by stench."

In short, stench was everywhere in those days, but were those smells actually *experienced* as stench at the time? There are definite indications that they were; in many countries, particularly in the eighteenth and nineteenth centuries, cleaning programs for streets, slaughterhouses, churches (in connection with the people buried there), houses, barracks, prisons and hospitals were conceived and implemented, the more so since stench was also held responsible for many ailments (Chapter 1).

Writers fill whole books with autobiographical data, but seldom discuss the smells of their past.[208] An exception to this was Gustave Flaubert, who in his correspondence with Louise Colet mentions inexhaustibly the smell of her slippers, dress, handkerchiefs and even her letters. Likewise the Dutch writer Maarten 't Hart, in whose story "The Burning Bush" a smell seems to influence the awakening of sexual feelings in a boy:

"Every year he looked forward to the autumn. When it came, he walked to the Schanshoofd, in order to bend forward into the water, where the hard stone head of the jetty gave way to the basalt slope. Then he could not only see little crabs scuttling away, but also smell something that was salty and dark and slightly decaying. But why could he only smell it in September? On that afternoon, too, he bent down as deeply as possible and stared at the stone of the quay wall, at the water with the swelling oil slicks, at the green, waving plumes of seaweed and the basalt blocks and inhaled the smell. The smell always made him sad, because he could only smell it for a moment, as though there were in that smell itself something sad, something like an unfulfilled desire for nostrils which will always be able to smell it, for a voice which could give it a name and for a place where it could be stored. [As the boy bends deeper, he is tugged at from the side by a girl. He tells her about the smell, and she wants to smell it, too.] "Give me your hand," she said, "hold me, because otherwise I'll fall." She bent over and hesitantly he took hold of her hand. "I can't smell anything," she said, "what am I supposed to smell?" "It's sharp and dark and it's a bit rotten," he said. "Dark," she said in surprise, "dark? Well, I can't smell anything." He didn't answer because something happened that took him completely by surprise. He smelled the smell for which he had been longing for a year stronger than ever. It was as though she made this smell suddenly more intense, but when she stood up in disappointment, he could still smell it and stayed sitting down, while she tried to free her hand from his. He was so absorbed in the smell all his muscles were tense, including the muscles of his hand, so she had to struggle to release her hand."

In the story "Mengelberg Interval," from the collection *The Winnowing Frame* by another Dutch writer, Ferdinand Bordewijk, the narrator smells the special smell of an unknown woman. "In the foyer amid the haze of cigarettes, the smell of black coffee and many different perfumes I smelled a smell. Thanks to a large nose with a well-developed sense of smell I smelled the smell before I saw anything. I have never smelled such a smell again. It wasn't perfume even in the most refined form—sweet, light and strange with something poisonous, dope-like about it. I resisted looking at the face of the woman who gave off this smell. I stood behind her until I was dizzy. Why wasn't everyone crowding around her and why wasn't she herself dizzy? I have never understood why not."

George Sand can also be mentioned in this connection.[209] "When she saw the blooming convolvuli, the mother said to me, 'Smell them, they smell like good honey; don't forget them!' So this is the first revelation of the sense of smell which I can recall, a link known to everyone but for me nevertheless inexplicable between memories and sensations; whenever I smell the smell of slender convolvuli, I always see in my mind's eye the place in the Spanish mountains at the side of the road where I picked these flowers for the first time."

Nevertheless, the sense of smell seldom plays an important part in recent literature. It is often demonstrated, though, that smells can activate memory. In Proust, the smell of a *petite madeleine* dipped into tea produces a feeling of euphoria. As the narrator wonders what the reason for this is, his memories of Combray, the place where he spent his youth, are evoked. His aunt Léonie gave him a piece of cake like that dipped in tea every Sunday morning when he went to say good morning to her in her bedroom. Confrontations with smells lead Proust to remember all kinds of experiences, some of which took place a very long time ago. Smells provoke him into a search for lost time, which is the title of his book.

The sixteenth-century philosopher Montaigne wrote an essay on smells. Montaigne considered himself a great smeller—supposedly because of his mustache, which retained smells from the air. On the basis of experience he notes that the best thing for a man is to be free of smells, particularly in the company of other people.

Women have better hygiene than men and so in his view come closer to the ideal. This is reminiscent of a remark by Plautus, who said that women smell particularly well when they are odorless.[210] Montaigne considered perfumes suspect, for they mask unpleasant smells and hence give a rosier impression than is justified. Smelling nice, according to Montaigne, is in fact synonymous with stinking, or as Martial said in antiquity, not without cynicism: "Under the ground the well-perfumed stink just as bad."[211]

Chapter 6

Odor-Driven Behavior

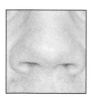 fter smells have been perceived via the olfactory organ and the signals have been assigned part of their meaning in the brain (rhinencephalon), the information is not left idle "upstairs." Generally the meaning of a smell is linked to information made available by other sensory systems. One difference between smell and the other senses, however, is that the ultimate interpretation of smell impressions takes place mainly in (and mainly affects) those parts of the brain connected with emotions, feelings and motivation (such as the amygdaloid nuclei in the limbic system, the hypothalamus and the right hemisphere). As a result, the sensation of smell leads quite often to a fairly direct behavioral response.[212] Precisely how such processes operate is still largely unclear, but that they do in fact take place is clear. Anyone smelling natural gas drops even the most interesting activity in order to do something about the danger. The smell of thiol and the awareness that the danger is threatening (via conditioning) have become linked.

Perception and Action

Generally, in the animal kingdom there are relationships between perceptual and behavioral abilities; one is often geared to the other. Perceiving something for perception's sake, as humans do in art or by way of recreation, is not useful or meaningful from a purely evolutionary point of view. The most important function of a sense is to ensure that the surroundings arc structured, usable information is obtained and appropriate behavior is activated in response. In other words, the senses must enable an animal to follow a *direction* in its actions; to survive, the animal must not be lost in a cacophony of sensory messages.

Frogs—to take one example of the coordination of perception and behavior—see only light and shadow and moving dots. The seeing of light and dark is necessary in order for the frog to be able to warm up and cool down; the dots direct the frog to the insects on which it lives. In this animal the link between perception and behavior is nearly perfect: a frog needs to know no more about its surroundings. This rigid, uncomplicated combination is less clearly present in higher animals. For example, carnivores appear to "know" that a predator is still around, even though it has disappeared from sight—a trait called "object permanence." Herbivores like cows and horses lack this ability. This difference is understandable: because grass does not creep away, no object permanence is needed.

Finally, human beings, who through cultural evolution have ensured that they create their own surroundings, are nowadays confronted with much more information than they can absorb (such as a thousand advertising messages a day, as well as countless meaningless traffic signs). Moreover, we absorb all kinds of information that is scarcely of any use to us (for example, the depressing scenes on television, wars, massacres, natural disasters). Therefore, for our own survival, we are well advised to ignore much information.[213]

Social Factors and Well-Being

Smells (whether or not we produced them) say something about the surroundings in which we find ourselves. Compared to the many images we absorb willingly or unwillingly every day, smells are "more assertive." Smells may have a directing influence on our actions, and often smells have a greater effect on our behavior than is generally thought.

As we have seen, smells are poorly "articulated" at the conscious level. In other words, we have no language, no clear grammar or syntax for this kind of information. Nevertheless, smells influence our behavior, often without our being aware of it. Olfactory information is processed mainly at the level of the cortex in the right hemisphere, a part of the brain that has little connection with language and in that respect functions "unconsciously" (at least so some researchers believe).[214] If the olfactory organ is stimulated through both nostrils, you could say that the left hemisphere reacts "intellectually" and the right mainly "emotionally." Moreover, the right hemisphere, as we noted previously, contains mainly crude motor programs; thus the smell perception of danger is generally followed by behavior in which the whole body is set in motion, as in flight reactions.

We shall look more closely at a number of physiological and social processes that are partly driven or affected by smells. A person's body odor can have physiological effects on other people, and apart from that, smells influence social behavior, interactions and relations between people, so their importance for social intercourse must not be underestimated (when Germans don't like someone, they say, *"Ich kann ihn nicht riechen"* (I can't [bear to] smell him); in Dutch we say that we can't stand the smell or sight of someone). There are also olfactory effects at a "higher level"—that is, in the social context. Think of smell pollution, the unpleasant smell in office buildings, the disruption of nature through the dominance of certain smells, but also the economically inspired use of smells to increase productivity and the impulse to buy.

In this context the individual's ability to control his environment is limited. The syndrome of sickness-causing office buildings in Europe, for example, is responsible for the financial loss of over a billion dollars annually, partly through a decline in productivity and absenteeism. These illness phenomena and complaints about the buildings in general are caused by a chronic "alarming" of the sense of smell by the stench that is normally there; unfortunately, the responsible people (architects, contractors, commissioning bodies) can seldom be convinced of this. Smells often have an alarm function: if you smell something, you want to know *what* you are smelling and *where* the smell is coming from. In a building like this, that is not possible; the cocktail is meaningless, it is everywhere, and it leads to a feeling of chronic stimulation and irritation.[215] This phenomenon is underestimated in part because test subjects have been asked to smell air samples under different circumstances. They are then inclined to say that the stink is not too bad. However, it makes a great deal of difference whether you smell the smell for just a moment or are exposed to it all day long, all the more so because adaptation to complex mixtures of smells is far from complete.[216]

In the outside air about 20 percent of the Dutch population turn out to have trouble with unpleasant smells. The aim is to halve this percentage by the year 2000, if we can believe the government. In the Rotterdam area alone, 6,500 complaints a year are recorded—twenty a day on average. Stench increases stress; some people say they become "raving mad" because of it. That is understandable. Such forms of stress require internal adaptation: we are obliged to take no notice of the unpleasant circumstances, in this case stench. It is well known that internal adaptation to stress is generally not good for one's health, in contrast to external adaptation, in which we change our environment (someone who is troubled by the noise of traffic closes the window). In addition, in the north of the Netherlands dozens of houses will probably be demolished because living in the vicinity of a processing factory for abattoir waste from pigs, cows, sheep and chickens has become intolerable.[217] It is striking that the objectively measurable stench has been reduced in recent years, yet the number of complaints is increasing. Perhaps people are becoming more aware of the growing problem of the environment, and they are more alert than they used to be.[218]

Synchronization of the Menstrual Cycle

In a strange physiological phenomenon, odors of female origin may bring about a synchronization of the menstrual cycle. Women who live in a residential group, share a room or are intimate friends eventually begin to menstruate around the same time. This synchronization is also found in many other mammals.[219] Of course it may be caused by correspondences in the day-night rhythm (circadian rhythm), lifestyle, eating habits, social interaction, work environment, age, etc., but synchronization also occurs when the women are initially very different in day-night rhythm, eating habits and age.[220] Consequently, it is suspected that a smell is responsible for the synchronization of the cycles or encourages it. This view was supported by the following experiment. Using gauze bandages, the armpit sweat of women with normal cycles was collected. Three times a week the upper lip of women with a very irregular cycle was rubbed with this substance. After four months, the cycles of all of the women had moved in the direction of the donor women (compared with women who had a normal cycle and who had been treated with a neutral gauze bandage dipped in an odorless solution).

Although these results seem unambiguous, there are some snags. For example, the experiment was not carried out in a double-blind way; both the donor and the receptor women (as well as the women who collected the sweat and rubbed it into the experimental women's lips) knew the point of the research. Even more important, the person conducting the experiment acted as a donor. Double-blind studies, however, have confirmed the results: female sweat deriving from regularly menstruating women can affect the cycles of other women.[221] Moreover, it is conceivable (albeit not essential for the findings) that the "synchronization substance" is absorbed not through the olfactory epithelium but through the skin.

Nevertheless, results must be treated with caution, because a number of confusing factors are involved. For example, it has been shown that the cycles of women living together who have no or scarcely any contact with men tend to become longer (the *Lee-Boot effect*), whereas the cycles of women who have quite a lot of contact with men—whether sexual or not—on average become slightly shorter.[222] The role smells play in this synchronization emerges indirectly from animal experiments. Dogs can distinguish menstruating women (particularly those in the second half of the menstrual cycle) from non-menstruating women on the basis of their body odor, probably because the body odor is at that time influenced by a considerable quantity of progesterone. Possibly this smell also has an (unconscious) effect on the behavior of people and on their hormonal economy.

Smell and Behavior

Smells influence our mood and motivation and hence also our behavior (the oracle at Delphi, according to tradition, put herself in the mood by inhaling the smell of burning laurel). These effects may take place with or without our knowledge, but an explicit appreciation and judgment, including an appropriate pattern of behavior, can be attached only to consciously experienced olfactory perceptions.

In general, smells may be experienced as negative, positive or neutral. If we react negatively to a smell, we are provoked to behavior that reduces the smell sensation: the source has to be avoided or the cause removed. If we react positively, we follow behavior that leads us to retain or intensify the olfactory sensation: the source of what we smell is approached or the cause of the smell retained. If we react neutrally, we do not care what happens to the smell or its source. We smell something, but the smell does not refer to anything we know or consider important; for that reason neutral smells are particularly suitable for making associations through conditioning (see Chapter 5, where we discussed the role of smell as a memory aid).

A few examples of this principle. When milk boils over and burns, three reactions are possible: leaving the house (avoiding the source), turning off the gas (removing the cause) or doing nothing. If the danger increases despite efforts to remove the cause, it is preferable to avoid the source by moving away. On the other hand, it is conceivable that the smell of the pizzeria around the corner leads us not to boil cabbage (to retain the cause of the smell) and to order a pizza with Gorgonzola (to approach the source).

Generally, however, things are much more complicated in practice, partly because the smell sensation can change or even turn into its opposite. One's mood, together with many bodily processes, determines whether one interprets a smell as positive or negative: a phenomenon known as alliesthesia (Chapter 5).[223] Everyone knows that the smell of a spicy meal is judged differently before eating than afterward. And a fervent vegetarian can become nauseous if you serve bacon for breakfast; for a carnivore it makes his day.

Consciously experienced striking smells generally have a warning function. Ask someone to list smells, and he or she will think mainly of unpleasant and penetrating smells. Pleasant or neutral smells are anchored less well in consciousness and memory. That is because such smells are, generally speaking, less associated with behavior, in contrast to smells connected with danger, which lead to a general reaction such as walking away or fleeing. It is beyond dispute that certain smells have direct effects on behavior. Even so, we also must be aware that in general there are great individual differences in the perception of smell and the appreciation of smell, and thus in any ensuing action. In other words: the olfactory system belongs to the brain's "software"; it is not rigid "hardware" which triggers compulsive or reflex-like reactions with a fixed pattern.

Our reactions to smells are often variable because the appreciation of smell is to a large extent acquired.[224] For example, we saw previously that children are fairly tolerant with regard to many smells; on the basis of experiences and through a process of punishment and reward they eventually develop preferences. Dislike or preference is not determined first and foremost by the smell itself, but by "operant conditioning," a form of learning that plays a large part in the life of humans and animals and in which behavior is shaped by rewarding and punishing. It is well known that young children have a tendency to eat the most awful things and, in contrast to animals, pay no attention to the smell.

According to many olfactory researchers no smell is innately unpleasant to human beings: in their eyes the olfactory system is a tabula rasa, a blank tablet. This view, however, is controversial, and linked to the eternal nature-nurture debate in biology and psychology—namely, whether qualities are genetically determined or are rooted in environmental factors such as upbringing. As often in this kind of opposition, the truth is generally somewhere in between. This also applies to smell. Studies suggest that newborn infants in perceiving smell even before their first feeding produce facial expressions that show many similarities to those of adults.[225] This fact indicates that in reactions to smells hereditary or even evolutionary factors may be involved. So the tabula rasa theory has to be qualified somewhat.

Although smell appreciation and associated behavior are heavily dependent on a person's upbringing and cultural background, from the very beginning the sense of smell can distinguish certain smells and assign meanings to them. Below, in a discussion of pheromones, we shall see that smells can evoke behavior without there being any appreciable learning process preceding it. Also, from research into the "olfactory bond" between mother and child, it will be seen that the view of the blank tablet requires qualification.

Smell and Interpersonal Behavior

Smells help to determine our social interaction. They can confirm and reinforce the links between relatives; they promote and intensify the contact between parents and children; and they mark the development and consolidation of social and even sexual relations. More than that, in experiments not only can we recognize our own smell, which accompanies us constantly and permeates our domestic surroundings, but this smell might also be of great importance for our feelings of well-being and safety and certainty. A strange house does not *smell* of us; partly as a result, we often feel slightly disoriented there. Perhaps this is one of the reasons why camping can be so nice: the tent smells familiar after just a few hours and so makes camping "fun." The bridal suite in an expensive hotel cannot compete with it. It has been said that astronauts were given domestic smells to take with them into space to prevent homesickness.[226]

In research into social behavior a distinction is made among interactions, relationships and structures.[227] If person A displays behavior focused on B, and B does something in respect to A, then there is an interaction between A and B. If that interaction turns out to influence the further course of contacts between these people, then A and B are in a relationship with each other. If such an interaction has no effect, then there is no relationship between A and B (for example, you have an interaction but no relationship with the train conductor when you show your ticket). If A and B are members of a group in which they have a definite position, then that relationship forms part of a social structure, which can be regarded as a network of relationships between individuals.

In discussing the influence of smells, biological and psychological meanings have to be weighed against each other. Smells that affect contacts in the general sense often have different effects than smells that help to maintain an existing social structure. In this context we will turn our attention to pheromones, substances important in the influencing of the behavior of other people in a relationship or in the creation of a mutual link between animals and human beings. In Chapter 7 we look at the role of perfumes and focus on the "olfactory passport" of human beings—namely, the individual aroma that each of us has. Olfactory passports are important in the formation and maintenance of a social network; they have a function in recognition and partly as a result of this the recognition socially of one's partner, children, relatives and peers.

Smell and Sex

In many animal species an intact olfactory organ is a necessary precondition for the displaying of sexual behavior. Various data confirm that smell also has some importance for human beings in this respect: the rhinencephalon has either direct or short links with systems in the brain and with parts of the endocrine system that are connected with eroticism and sex. In addition, there are close connections between the olfactory organ, the hypothalamus (which among other things is essential for the expression of emotions, the swelling of the genitalia, and orgasm), the hypophysis and the glands that produce sex hormones.

These are designated the "naso-genital alliance": smells influence sexual arousal and activity, and sexual behavior is reflected in the perception and processing of smells, possibly through changes in hormonal balance.[228] The lines of influence are probably as follows: hormones—smells (such as body smells and the pheromones to be discussed below)—sex—hormones—sense of smell. Men and women appear to have slightly different olfactory "neural circuits" in their brains, and this distinction is responsible for differences between the sexes in the erotic sphere.[229] Finally, animals and human beings alike use the nose to investigate others' genitalia.

To a certain extent we can find traces of the "naso-genital alliance" in everyday life, in language and in all kinds of attitudes. The size of the nose is often associated with the degree of virility. In antiquity adulterous men were punished with amputation of the nose, a practice described in Virgil's *Aeneid.* Some centuries ago doctors even believed that they could tell whether girls were still virgins by feeling their noses. Abnormalities in a nose, too, were thought to be caused by excessive sexual activity; chronic colds were supposed to indicate frequent sexual intercourse.[230]

One possible basis for these ideas is the following. The internal structure of the nose shows a certain correspondence with the swelling organs in the penis. This may lead a man to sneeze at the sight of an attractive woman; the beginning of an erection often leads to a swelling and a rise in the temperature in the nasal epithelium (the naso-genital reflex). In women, too, there are links between the nose and the genitals: nosebleeds are supposed to be connected with menstruation. This is not totally absurd: in rhesus monkeys it has been observed that the swelling and reddening of the ano-genital area is linked with the swelling of the olfactory mucous membrane.

Pheromones: General Remarks

Animals produce three sets of odors that affect the behavior of other animals: *kairomones*, *allomones* and *pheromones*. A kairomone attracts animals of other species; for example, the tsetse fly tends to be attracted to the smell of the buffalo. An allomone repels animals of other species, as a skunk does. Odors with which an animal lures others of the same species to engage in a certain kind of behavior—or even forces them to—are called pheromones. For a substance to be called a pheromone, it must have an effect even in a very small concentration. Pheromones can be compared with hormones, with one difference being that they assert their influence outside the body. The similarity with hormones is partly a matter of names: pheromone is a contraction of the Greek words for "carry" (*pherein*) and "provoke" or "stimulate" (*horman*). Pheromones do not always produce an immediately apparent reaction, however. For example, a distinction is made between pheromones that affect the endocrine system (which produces sex hormones), pheromones that facilitate physiological changes of various kinds (*primer pheromones*) and pheromones that directly provoke a certain behavior in the observer (*releaser pheromones*).[231]

Pheromones often play a part in sexual behavior, but they can also have a communicative function. Flies leave behind an olfactory trace for the benefit of other flies in places where food is to be found; ants, besides sex pheromones, also have "trail-following pheromones" with an "altruistic" function; schools of fish may stay together because of smells. Greenflies and termites in peril secrete an alarm pheromone, which warns their fellow creatures to avoid a particular environment, and some species of fish emit shock pheromones. Many other animal species mark their territory with smells, behavior that also has a communicative function.

Such discoveries have led researchers to trace the structural formulas of pheromones, and these formulas become the basis of synthetic products used in combating insects. The release of pheromone does not always turn out well for their producer, however. For example, it is possible that an animal that releases lots of sex pheromones is so besieged by its fellows that it does not actually achieve reproduction.

Even in the plant kingdom one sees phenomena that show similarities with the three types of substances mentioned above; they are often warning signals or defense mechanisms. If a willow is plagued by certain insects, it warns other willows with a special scent; these willows then produce a substance that deters insects.[232] When the leaves of the white clover leaf are damaged, they produce poisonous cyanide, which functions in the manner of an allomone. In such circumstances the tomato produces a substance that disturbs the digestion of insects, and a certain Mexican flower (*Ageratum houstonianum*) upsets the hormonal balance of attacking insects. Corn plants give off kairomone-like substances. Plants attacked by caterpillars produce odors that attract creeping wasps; the wasps exterminate the caterpillars by laying eggs in their bodies.

Discoveries in Insects

The term *pheromone* came into use in the late 1950s among entomologists. The odors concerned have been known for much longer, in mammals as well as insects, and even in single-cell organisms pheromone-like substances can be found.[233] There was a need, however, for a term for species-specific reactions to a particular odor.

The operation of pheromones is most pronounced in insects. Pheromones may direct behavior in mammals such as rats, but they do not always provoke a reflexive, compulsive reaction. (An exception to this rule is the phenomenon of lordosis in pigs, about which more below.)

The most suggestive attractive power of a pheromone has been found in the silkworm moth *Bombyx mori.* The female secretes a substance, bombykol, which the male recognizes many kilometers away (Chapter 1).[234] With its relatively large antennae— equipped with olfactory receptors sensitive only to bombykol— he is able to trace the female.[235] The female depends on the male's capacity to detect her; she has much smaller antennae and can scarcely smell him even if he is in her immediate vicinity. This does not mean that the female leads an odorless existence: she makes excellent use of her antennae to find a suitable place to lay her eggs.

Von Frisch, the discoverer of the "language of bees," also known as the bee dance, investigated the significance of chemical signals in the life of the honeybee.[236] The queen bee is recognized by her subjects through her distinctive smell. The worker bees form a circle around her, so that she can lay her eggs at her leisure. Entomologists call this phenomenon "court behavior." The queen's palette of smells enables the others to locate and·identify her in a beehive. That is of great importance, for the queen is not much larger than an ordinary worker bee. That "court behavior" is reinforced through smell is clear from the following experiment. Take a worker bee who is a member of the queen's circle, and who therefore carries a little of her aroma, and put her in a box in which worker bees have been isolated for hours away from the queen. After a while the worker bee is treated as a princess by the others.[237] This suggests that the other workers' behavior in relation to the queen is caused by a pheromone, and other experiments confirm this. The pheromone manifests itself not only as an odor; worker bees also touch and lick the queen, the combination of smell and taste ensuring that the pheromone is spread through the honeycomb. It turns out that this pheromone also suppresses the development of the ovaries of worker bees (a *primer* function of the pheromone; see above), so that the queen remains the only fertile female. If the queen dies, the inhibiting effect of the substance disappears, and several larvae develop into potential successors. The same pheromone also stimulates the drones to accompany the queen on her flight (a *releaser* function).

Pheromones in Mammals and Human Beings

Drawing on pheromone research in insects, researchers looked for similar substances in mammals and humans. It soon became clear that the behavior-specific and compulsive action of pheromones found in insects is rarely if ever found in that form in mammals. The behavior of mammals is much more complex and flexible, and is driven by a greater quantity and variety of sensory information.[238] Moreover, the activity of higher mammals is more variable, as insects have virtually only instincts—*adapted*, but not generally *adaptable*, behavior. An example is the creeping wasp, which inspects a cavity before putting its prey inside. If someone moves the prey a fraction in the meantime, the wasp puts the object back at the edge of the cavity and inspects the hole again. It will repeat this procedure ad infinitum if necessary. In short, insects, unlike mammals, do not learn; their behavior is prescribed in a compulsory and reflex way. (The difference in adaptability of behavior between insects and lower animals and mammals, however, is gradual and not categorical; so we must be careful in drawing facile conclusions.)

Because of the complexity of their behavior, in discussing mammals one usually does not refer to *releaser pheromones* but to *signaling pheromones*, a term indicating that the odors involved have (only) a signaling function in relation to specific behavior. Without supplementary stimuli from other sensory systems the reactions will not be displayed. In other words, signaling pheromones are odors involved in certain (sexual) behavior in mammals, but that behavior depends on supplementary communications via other sensory channels. The operation of *primer pheromones* is also less clear in mammals than in insects. For these reasons certain researchers want to abolish or drastically limit the use of the term *pheromone* in reference to mammals.[239] Yet it is clear that, as in insects, smell and reproduction are closely connected in mammals: removal of the bulbus olfactorius leads to sterility in female mice. Strangely enough, that is not the case with males.[240]

Pheromone research in mammals and humans has concen-

trated on two kinds of substances: *androstenes* and *copulines*—
that is, male and female pheromones, respectively. In females both
kinds of substances are found. The discovery of 5α-androst-16-en-
3α-ol, or *androstenol* for short, in sweat and urine, particularly of
men (specifically in the armpits), and of *estradiol*, a fatty substance found in the vaginal secretion of monkeys, stirred a tidal
wave of questions and hypotheses. The testing of these showed a
number of defects, but that has improved over time.[241]

Quite apart from the question of whether there is a specific
human sex pheromone, some time ago it was suggested that such
substances influence our actions in general.[242] That suspicion was
prompted by the sexual revolution of the 1960s, which, incidentally, highlighted the importance of the sense of smell. For example, Freud, following on the views of Fliess, observed that the
unlimited appreciation of bodily odors is strongly suppressed in
modern society and that the neglect of them might lead to mental
disturbances. Wilhelm Reich can also be mentioned in this context; his works were very popular in the 1960s.

It is obvious that shaving one's armpits has a negative effect
on the retention and spread of pheromone-like substances possibly
present in sweat, as does the use of deodorants and deodorizing
shower and bath soaps, which often contain antibacterial substances. Because bacteria living in the armpits play an important
part in the production of pheromone-like compounds, a deodorant
may drastically damage one's personal aroma. A possible result of
depilation is that men are regarded with somewhat less interest
by women; conversely, a woman's use of a deodorant may lead
men to show less interest in her.

A speculative hypothesis on armpit sweat is as follows. When
man began walking upright he smelled less, because most odors
hover just above ground level. In those circumstances the body
odor of a fellow human being can be properly perceived only if
the most important source is placed "high" in the body—namely,
in the armpits, or not too far from the nose.

There is no shortage of anecdotes about the influence of human odor.[243] A young man clutched a handkerchief in his sweating
armpit while dancing and subsequently offered it to the lady, who,

the story goes, found that its smell stimulated her erotically. Or girls sometimes carried halves of apples in their armpits while dancing, then offered them to their male partners, apparently with a similar result. Conversely, Ovid, in *The Art of Love*, recommends that one not allow any repulsive goat-like smell to arise in the armpits.[244]

Female Pheromones

When a mare in heat and a stallion are together and the stallion investigates the mare's ano-genital area with interest, she commonly urinates. He sometimes puts his nose into the stream of her urine or inhales its smell. Subsequently he raises his head and parts his lips. This behavior is called "flaring," or the flehmen response, from the German word for cajoling or coaxing.[245] Flaring occurs commonly in herbivores of both sexes; it is connected with the vomeronasal organ (Chapters 2, 4), which is a sac that makes a connection between the oral and nasal cavities through a channel between the incisor teeth. The receptors present in this organ assess (via the investigation of the urine) the degree of heat or receptivity.[246] Flaring, in short, means inhaling certain smells connected with sexual behavior.

This organ can be damaged or removed altogether without disastrous results, but in inexperienced animals removal probably leads to a disturbance of sexual behavior.[247] There are good reasons to assume that the vomeronasal organ is involved in imprinting processes in the sexual field, as can be deduced as well from anatomical links of the nerve fibers with the limbic system.[248] It is striking that there is no feedback from the limbic system to the vomeronasal organ; the information goes in one direction only (as was said, in man the vomeronasal organ degenerates during embryonic development).

Apart from their apparent sexual signaling function, the pheromones in urine and vaginal fluid perform other functions in animals. The sexual maturation of female mice is delayed, for example, when they grow up in a group consisting only of female mice; obviously the presence of male pheromones and female sexual development are connected.[249] Conversely, within a few moments the urine of a female in estrus is able to produce marked fluctuations in the hormonal balance of the male (in particular, noradrenaline and the luteinizing hormone LH shoot upward after a confrontation). In humans these kinds of phenomena have not yet been investigated, but a similar principle applies to other animals. For example, if estradiol, a substance found in the vaginal fluid of rhesus monkeys, is applied to the vaginal region of females whose ovaries have been removed, the sexual interest of males is revived; if the nostrils of the male monkey are subsequently blocked, then interest declines markedly.[250]

A strange thing happens with mice. When mice mate, pregnancy almost always results. If after mating the male mouse is removed and replaced by another male, then the female generally does not produce any young. The strange smell of the other male leads to premature abortion, as it were. Clearly the smell of a male mouse affects the hormonal balance of the female.

It is well known that volatile chemical substances of female origin play some part in the courtship, mating and pregnancy of animals. In order to provide the isolated male pheromones (androstenes) known from structural formulas with female counterparts, the collective name "copulines" was proposed.[251] These are substances that (as the name implies) are thought to play a part in stimulating sexual activity in males of the same species. The effect of copulines on human behavior, however, has turned out to be rather hypothetical; for example, men generally regard vaginal odor as unpleasant. Yet Henry III remained in love with Mary of Clèves all his life after smelling the scent of her underwear (pheromones?) and Goethe admitted that he had stolen one of Mrs. von Stein's corsets in order to smell it at his leisure.[252]

An estradiol-like substance found in human vaginal secretions was consequently—expectantly—called human copuline, and a research project was set up to test its operation.[253] Sixty-two couples participated. The breasts of the women were rubbed with copuline, perfume, alcohol or water. The results provided no proof for the hypothesis: copuline had no discernible influence on sexual activity. This research is open to criticism, however.

The couples were used to going to bed with each other quite frequently (on average, more than twice a week), so arguably the operation of copuline (for the man) was of little importance.[254] In addition, each couple had to use one of the four substances in a random order—for example, night 1 (copuline), night 3 (alcohol), night 5 (copuline), night 7 (water), night 9 (perfume)—so the copuline applied on night 1 may have kept working till night 3. It would have been more sensible to administer a particular substance for a number of nights in succession. In short, the existence of a female sex pheromone in human beings cannot be excluded, but such a conclusion cannot yet be drawn.

In a different experiment,[255] test subjects were asked to look at photographs of boys and girls and describe them in accordance with a number of criteria. They did so under two conditions: once when a relatively neutral odor was disseminated, and once with the (unpleasant) vaginal odor of monkeys. With assessment criteria such as "reliability," "cheerfulness" and suchlike, it made no difference what smell the test subjects had inhaled. With the notions "sexy" and "shy," however, there was a difference. Under the influence of the vaginal odor, boys and girls alike found the photos of girls more sexy. The boys also mentioned "less shy." The experiment seems to indicate that vaginal odors of monkeys can affect our judgment of other people, and affect males more strongly than females. We don't know, however, whether this phenomenon affects (sexual) behavior.

Another unanswered question is why partners who are having conflicts in their relationship often complain about each other's bodily odors. It may be that they have "incompatible" smells, or it may be that they attribute their difficulties to smells. Yet we know that mice prefer to mate with other mice whose urine smells slightly different from theirs; the smell of the urine is supposed to say something about the genetic makeup of the partner.[256]

Male Pheromones

There are a number of indications for the existence of male pheromones. Androstenes are found in small concentrations in male

armpit sweat (and, strangely enough, particularly in December[257])
and in moderation in saliva and urine. The concentrations vary
widely from person to person, and only sexually mature males
secrete these substances in significant amounts. The production
of androstenes increases with sexual excitement. Mature women
also produce traceable quantities of male pheromones, but on
average only one-fifth of the amount typically produced by men
—although, women, incidentally, can secrete as many or more
androstenes than the average man.

Again, the highest concentration of androstenes is found in the
armpits.[258] Sweat itself is odorless, but bacteria like *Corynebacte-
rium* and *Proteus vulgaris* convert certain chemical compounds
into androstenes and other substances, which often produce a
pungent smell (some people suffer from *bromidrosis*, an abnormal
sweaty smell, which may be linked to excessive quantities of these
microorganisms). Thus far four androstenes have been identified
in sweat, such as androstenone and the derived alcohol androstenol. The odorless base of androstenone is probably testosterone,
the male sex hormone. Other substances too, such as cholesterol,
pregnenolone, androstenone and dehydroxy-epi-androsterone,
probably play roles in the production of androstenes.[259]

Do we appreciate androstenes? The situation is rather confusing. For example, androstene has a urine-like smell, which most
people find disgusting, whereas androstenol smells of musk and
most people find it pleasant. As the concentration is increased, so
does the subject's dislike of androstene, but as we saw in Chapter 3, in a mixture an unpleasant smell can be masked or a pleasant
one reinforced.

Many people turn out to be anosmic for androstenes; for example, almost half the population cannot perceive the smell of
androstenone. There are indications that genetic factors may be
connected with this inability.[260] Anosmia for androstenone, however, does not mean that there is never a *reaction* to the odor. It
has been shown that the electrical resistance of the skin (the galvanic skin response, or GSR, an indicator, for example, for alertness) can drop sharply after an encounter with androstenone,
particularly when the odor is not consciously perceived.[261] This

fall is an indication of a general rise in activity in the emotional field, too. If the smell is experienced consciously and is found to be pleasant, such a fall also occurs; if the odor is found to be unpleasant, however, then the GSR does not change perceptibly. These are remarkable phenomena, as they show a difference between the effects of conscious and unconscious perceptions of smell. With unconscious perception the general bodily level of activity increases, but if the perception penetrates consciousness, the reaction then becomes highly dependent on the appreciation of the smell. It follows from this that such a smell can influence the physical and mental condition in various ways, depending on the concentration. On the basis of these data we can suspect that smells can steer our behavior in a particular direction without our noticing it.

It has emerged from experiments that the galvanic skin response to androstenone is less pronounced in women than in men. This is less surprising than it seems, because much depends on whether the test subject can *name* the odor. Women are generally more capable of naming smells, so that anosmia for androstenone (in men) may be partly due to their lack of a "label." As a result, men may be inclined to deny having any perception of the smell, a phenomenon which in them is linked with a relatively strong GSR. After an arbitrary name was given to androstenone, a number of anosmic test subjects turned out to be remarkably well able to smell it (and the strength of the GSR dropped sharply). A conscious experience therefore seems to have an inhibiting effect on physical reactions. In short, it seems that androstenone functions like a pheromone, provided that it is not smelled consciously or is spread in subtle quantities. In general, women find the smell of androstenone less pleasant than men do, but whether women are more sensitive to this substance—in the sense that their threshold value is lower—has not been established.[262] In general, we can say that the smell of androstenes is unpleasant, but in a mixture with other substances it might seem quite the contrary. And as we saw, a conscious assessment is certainly not the only factor that determines the effect of androstenes.

How is the behavior of animals (mammals) influenced by these substances? In pigs, androstenes are used in order to determine the fertility of the sow. In the past, the farmer sat astride the sow and tried to push her forward. If the sow resisted, it was supposed that she was in heat. This method turned out to be unreliable, since only half of sows in estrus display that behavior. When confronted with a boar, a sow in estrus becomes motionless, rounds her back and pricks up her ears, an action which is called lordosis, or the mating stance. In our age of artificial insemination, this stance has fallen into disuse, but a "natural diagnostic technique" has been developed. The sow's snout is sprayed with an aerosol substance containing androstenone and androstenol. If the animal is in heat, this substance produces lordosis.[263] This method has been used successfully with sheep and cows as well. The odor of a bull also lowers the age at which a heifer can calve: the odor accelerates the onset of puberty in the heifer—a principle that we previously saw in mice and that also applies to many other animals.

Before one protests against the use of such an aerosol out of concern for the welfare of sows, consider that sows find androstenes very pleasant. Not only do they associate this odor with the boar; they also use the desire for androstenes to find tasty morsels. Sows, for example, have a very fine nose for truffles. A truffle is a mushroom with a tuber which is formed under the ground, often at the foot of oak trees (so-called truffle oaks), and sows can smell truffles a meter or more deep. This ability is due mainly to their extreme sensitivity to pheromones, for truffles contain a high concentration of androstenes.[264] For many human beings, too, truffles—partly because of the pheromones in the mixture?—are a delicacy. The question remains whether human beings are also influenced by androstenes in their behavior.

In one controversial study, the effects of copuline and androstenol were investigated in assessing applicants for an administrative post at a university.[265] The members of the appointment committee were given masks such as those used by surgeons, on the pretext that their facial expressions should have as little influence as possible on the behavior of the candidates. Some masks were odorless, others impregnated with androstenol or copuline; the committee members, however, were unaware. Androstenol, it turned out, led female committee members to assess male candidates more positively, whereas copuline and androstenol led the men on the committee to respond more negatively to the women applicants. The effects were not convincing or spectacular, though, and the masks produced a good deal of hilarity, which probably did not benefit the validity of the assessments. Moreover, some other smell in the reception area may have affected the results.[266] The masks containing copuline and androstenol would have distorted this smell, whereas the odorless masks would have let it flow unimpeded.

Another experiment showed that women in photographs were found more attractive by subjects of both sexes if the subjects wore masks containing androstenol.[267] But it is doubtful that the smell of androstenol always has a marked influence on someone's "emotional" judgment. In reading an erotic story, test subjects wearing masks treated with androstenol entered the same values for their degree of pleasure or sexual stimulation as did subjects wearing odorless masks or masks sprayed with rose water.[268] Again, wearing such a thing on one's face makes the experiment unnatural, so the data may not be very significant. It would be more sensible to investigate the effects of such odors without the test subjects having any suspicion of the intention of the experiment.

In another experiment, chairs in a dentist's waiting room were sprayed with various concentrations of androstenone (which is related to androstenol, but is less stable chemically: androstenone is quite quickly converted into androstenol).[269] Women patients used those chairs more often, while men avoided them. The effect was most marked for the chairs sprayed with relatively low concentrations, which is consistent with our observations about physical influences of smells either unnoticed or scarcely noticed. Women, too, avoided the chairs sprayed with a high concentration of androstenone, suggesting that these substances work particularly when the quantities used are subtle. In a similar experiment conducted in a theater,[270] a number of chairs treated with androstenone were occupied mainly by women. Incidentally, more programs from "androstene seats" were taken home, and the experiment disturbed the menstrual cycles of a number of the theater's female employees.

Nevertheless, we must not be too quick to conclude that women are simply attracted by the smell of such substances. An experiment on the campus of a university in California strikes a cautionary note.[271] Men's toilets sprayed with a smell of androstenol were used up to 80 percent less than previously. When ladies' toilets were sprayed, there was no difference in use: they were not made either more attractive or less attractive by the odor of androstenol. The duration of the observation was a week, which seems to have been sufficient time for the students to develop a preference. Even so, it might have been more sensible to observe behavior over a longer period, since the sensitivity to androstenol fluctuates considerably in women.

Research has also been conducted into the link between mood and androstenol in various phases of the menstrual cycle.[272] Female students of about twenty years of age were asked to put a drop of androstenol mixed with alcohol on their upper lip every morning after washing; another group applied a placebo containing only alcohol. None of the students were taking any contraceptive pills. They were asked to indicate their mood every day along the axes aggressive-submissive, happy-depressed, lively-listless, seductive-rejecting, and good humored-quickly irritated. The influence of androstenol was significant only in the aggressive-submissive category: androstenol led to fewer feelings of aggression, particularly around the time of ovulation. In that situation the students who used androstenol felt more "amenable" or submissive than those who had received the placebo. Although a submissive feeling is not the same as the immobilization reflex in sows, a certain relationship with the lordosis phenomenon may not be too far-fetched. It also emerged from this study that the students felt most depressed during menstruation.[273] This change of mood, however, was not linked with a change in self-image or in any of the other categories mentioned: the students did not consider themselves less lively, less sexy or more quickly irritated during menstruation.

Possibly such factors as the small size of the sample (eighteen women) and the large differences in the test results may have produced a masking effect.

Do male pheromones affect the length of the menstrual cycle? On the basis of what we know about the behavior of animals, such a substance has a certain effect on the duration and regularity of the cycle—as seen in the theater experiment.[274] In rodents, ovulation can be stimulated by having the animal smell the odor of the male's urine.[275] In human beings, the length of the cycle shifts more toward the average (that is, toward 29.5 plus or minus 3 days), the more time women spend with men, particularly if there is a fairly steady pattern in sexual activity—although if it is a matter of smells, cuddling would be sufficient.[276]

In order to investigate whether a pheromone is involved, researchers studied the effects of male armpit sweat on the menstrual cycle, this time with the necessary control measures (the aim of the study was not revealed to the test subjects).[277] Fifteen women with cycles shorter than 26 or longer than 32 days took part in the experiment. During three cycles, they applied male sweat extract to their upper lip three times a week without any significant influence on the cycle. Among the women who had contact with men not at all or less than once a week, the effects were significant. So there are reasons for excluding women who have relatively frequent contact with men from these kinds of experiments: they undergo the influence of male sweat more or less permanently. Nevertheless, it is strange that precisely those women often show a divergent cycle length.

Do Pheromones Have a Function in Humans?

According to biology, not much happens "for no reason" (apart from, it is said, the directionless process of evolution itself); all possible means are deployed in the struggle for existence. If something pleasant is happening (such as sexual contact), then the pleasure is in the service of biological necessity. If mating were generally a painful event, we would not go to bed with each other anymore, and without artificial insemination our species would soon die out. Although reproduction is not necessary for an individual to have a meaningful life, from a biological point of view we must ensure the transfer of genes, a.k.a. behavioral possibilities. We can do this indirectly, of course, looking after our nieces and nephews, who share a quarter of their genes with us.[278]

Our existence is not just a matter of biology and evolution, however. Unlike most animals, we create a large part of our environment: houses, clothing, schools, libraries, trades, art, science. This creative process has its own dynamism, a cultural evolution that is essential for our continued existence. Human beings, then, reproduce in two ways: physically and through the transfer of *information.* As regards the former, biologists believe that every living being tries to achieve the greatest possible degree of reproductive success. This view contains an infamous piece of circular reasoning: to the question why and in what respect one organism is more "fit" (that is, better adapted) than another, people usually refer to the fact that the one displays more reproductive success than the other, and the response to the question "Why is that?" is that the animal is more "fit." This tautological line of thought occurs in countless disheartening variations; some researchers have tried to break through the circle by using "function" and "adaptation" in a broader sense, without being too indebted to the reproduction argument.[279]

This is not to say that it is meaningless to ponder the adaptive or survival value of pheromones. Without an "ultimate analysis" —an explanation in terms of values that are decisive within the process of evolution and to which selection can attach—making a "proximate analysis" (explaining the physiological operation of pheromones) can be difficult. In other words, the evolutionary significance we assign to pheromones in part determines how we interpret the effects they appear to have here and now. What evolutionary significance do we assign to them, then? What is the advantage or disadvantage of the use of pheromones in light of reproduction? There are different ideas about this.

It is not possible to see when women are fertile. In other female mammals (such as monkeys), swelling is observable and/or the female (such as dogs) emit a specific smell. According to some researchers, the "hidden" character of ovulation in humans is a result of our species' more and more strongly developed self-consciousness in the course of evolution.[280] In a sense, they argue, our self-consciousness could be a danger to reproduction. We know that bearing and bringing up children is a painful and difficult matter. In order to prevent the extinction of the species, natural selection has led to sex being pleasurable for us, but also to sex having relatively unpredictable consequences. That combination ensures that human beings will not find it easy to "plan" reproduction. According to this view we have both intelligent and opportunistic characteristics, and we particularly keep our self-interest in view. Given the investment that has to be made to bear, nurse and bring up a child, we are not easily induced to reproduce. In order to produce a new generation, according to this line of reasoning, there has to be a "hard core" of relatively autonomously functioning physical and social processes that prevent us from dying out.

The hidden ovulation fits into this line of thought, as does the lack of a specific mating period in man. A "disadvantage" of the latter is that in a statistical sense we have to copulate often in order to bring about a pregnancy. From a biological-evolutionary point of view, however, we must be tempted to mate immediately after ovulation, when the chance of fertilization is greatest. The emission of a specific, irresistible odor—in short, a pheromone—fits into this scenario. In order to increase sexual activity around the time of ovulation, the system is regulated by a process of which we remain largely unconscious. This reduces the chance of our trying to suppress our impulses; a consciously executed sexual act, after all, leads us to start seeing all kinds of snags and risks.[281]

This line of reasoning seems rather farfetched: on the evolutionary time scale, self-consciousness is probably of relatively recent date. The process of natural selection no doubt required much more time to promote the subtle function of pheromones we have described; moreover, neither human beings nor animals are (or ever were) very well able to link events a long way apart in time (namely, copulation and birth). In short, is it not much more plausible to assert that the development of self-consciousness is *not* at odds with reproduction and enduring pain?

Another line of reasoning is the following.[282] Pheromones probably have such a disadvantageous effect in man that their operation has virtually disappeared. Hidden ovulation, it is argued, came about because of a change in the social structure of our distant ancestors. It is assumed that these human beings lived in small groups around a family with an adult male and one or more adult females (which we still see among apes, such as gorillas and gibbons). In those circumstances it was important that the female made it clear when she is fertile through swellings and/or smells; a species with a large number of "missed chances" would soon be eliminated by natural selection.

The situation changed at the end of the Miocene period, when, as a result of climatological changes, humanoids moved into the savannas, an area that also attracted large numbers of grazing animals. The only way of killing such large animals was cooperative hunting. As a result, man was obliged to live in larger groups, while because of the value of the parents' investment in their descendants, the monogamous (or, incidentally, polygamous) bond had to be maintained. In those circumstances "public" ovulation came under pressure. In the larger living unit, after all, the woman had more contact with men, so that a check on her loyalty became difficult; moreover, the number of potential fathers could become so large that no one man would be prepared to look after the child. That is a serious matter: faithfulness is important for the investment in the next generation; it would be in the interest of the woman for the man to share the food he has won with her and the children, and in the interest of the man that the food should reach his wife and children and not others. Natural selection, then, might have promoted hidden ovulation and a tendency to sharply reduce or deprive of meaning smells which betray ovulation.

Of these two accounts, with lots of speculation and presuppositions, the latter explanation is rather more elegant, because it takes account of such factors as the slow tempo of the evolutionary process. According to it, it was in man's interest for pheromones to be taken out of their original context and be given a neutral or innocent meaning. We can observe something similar today: a woman who smells nice will be perhaps treated in a more friendly way by both men and women, but one does not feel one-self attracted will-lessly and defenselessly to such a person. In other words: we are able to sublimate the meaning of a smell: its compulsive character has gone. We shall return to this question in discussing the role of perfumes.

These explanations focus on the lack of importance of female pheromones, but there are indications that human beings do have quite active male pheromones. What is the reason for that asymmetry? Rather than concluding that female pheromones have a subtle but nevertheless important function, we can try to devise a simpler (if no less speculative) line of reasoning.[283]

Where there is marked sexual dimorphism in the animal kingdom, one often sees harem formation—the red deer, the zebra, the baboon. The males must keep constant watch on the females, and must drive away attackers. A pheromone that attracts females while deterring other males might come in handy in such circumstances. Conversely, it must be in the interest of a female in the harem to secrete smells that signal a change in her condition—a repulsive smell when she is not in estrus, an attractive smell when she is. The result: the harem keeper will approach the female only when there is some point to his doing so. An example: lion monkey females "mark" most when they are pregnant—a useful behavior if the odor has a sexually inhibiting effect on the male (nothing is known about this, though).

However, sexual contact when there is marked sexual dimorphism is not always without risks. Even when the male and the female are equally strong, sex can harm one or the other. Courtship behavior often has an aggressive component (if necessary, sublimated in a love bite), but sometimes things go wrong, as with drakes, who—in a gang rape of sorts—can literally drown a female.

In humans this function of pheromones determined by sexual dimorphism may still exist in a weakened form. Men are on average heavier, stronger, quicker and more aggressive than women; nevertheless, they have to do their best to put women in a "mellow" mood. The upshot is that men are well advised to produce pleasant smells in order to attract women. The theater experiment and the experiment in the dentist's waiting room are consistent with this view.

This line of reasoning follows on from the fact that our ancestors originally lived in small groups. Gorillas and orangutans still do, and there are "bachelor groups" of males and solitary wandering males. The females remain mostly in their family group, unless a male is able to "hijack" one of them. In that case it is vital for the male not to stink or show aggressive behavior; possibly the female is mellowed somewhat by androstenes, so that she is prepared to accept male company.

Since human beings no longer generally live in harems, there is no compelling reason for the man to continue to please a woman with odors once he has won her. This means that pheromones have become anachronisms, vestiges from the time when we still lived on the savannas. Because these substances have not completely lost their significance for man's functioning, the production of them is not really obstructed by natural selection. Yet female pheromones contain a certain danger, since they betray whether ovulation is in progress. For that reason female pheromones over time may have been increasingly selected out of existence, and perhaps the male capacity to detect such substances has been increasingly suppressed.

But that is not the end of the story: it might be in women's interest to *inhibit* men's advances with the help of repellent odors. An attractive odor, after all, might make the woman the target of undesired suitors. Perhaps the use of perfume by women is connected with this, in that perfumes function as "masking" smells for pheromone-like substances. By this line of reasoning, women use perfume in order to be considered *unattractive* sexually.

A second implication of this reasoning is that perfumes for men today fit particularly into "courtship behavior," and are used in order to "pull" a woman. Once the relationship has been established, the man need not repeat this behavior but can relapse into his old and familiar smell regime, even if it pleases his woman only moderately. Biologically, however, it is in women's interest to attach herself to the man even after pregnancy so as to ensure his care for the next generation. Perhaps that is why women continue using perfume: in order to please the man generally or at least not repel him.

Chapter 7

Perfumes and
Olfactory Passports

We saw that our body odors can influence other people's behavior to some extent (as in the theater experiment). Smells also turn out to have some effect on our assessments of others, with rational considerations sometimes being relegated to a secondary position (as in the job application experiment). In view of these influences of smells on our behavior it is conceivable that people who believe that they give off unpleasant or telltale smells should want to do something to keep these from being smelled by others, even if there is no biological reason to mask those smells.

Of course, the impulse to hide certain smells and the uncertainty evoked by smelling particularly strange (that is, unfamiliar) body odors are to a large extent culturally determined. We do not want to be treated in too personal a way in public; after all, nothing is as personal as your body odor. In order to "keep your distance" the obvious thing to do is to replace your body odor with an "anonymous" lotion, aftershave or perfume. It is quite understandable that those fragrances should sometimes contain ingredients very similar to the components of body odors: we do not want to be *too* alienated from our familiar smell.[284]

According to various researchers, then, perfumes, particularly in women, have a certain protective role. We saw in the previous chapter why that might be the case: it is conceivable that long ago women had a biological interest in keeping their ovulation hidden. According to the theory of evolution, the process of natural selection would have encouraged the body's production of masking substances; and if those masking substances are not yet present, a woman might look in her environment for substances to mask a body odor which indicates that she is fertile.

Perfumes in the Past

This sexually protective function appears to play no significant role at the present time. A few centuries ago, it did to a certain extent, which gave rise to heated discussions.[285]

According to many people, women who used perfume were suspect because those perfumes were thought to betray ambitions in the marriage market. "The tender smell of marjoram which is exuded by a virgin is milder, more intoxicating than all the perfumes of Arabia put together," one moralist wrote. Indiscreet courting was to be condemned; the task of the sense of smell was at most to awaken desire without jeopardizing honor.

Others believed that you could not perfume yourself heavily enough, since with perfumes the miasmas in the surrounding air could be neutralized (Chapter 1). For analogous reasons gravediggers were advised to carry wads of cotton wool soaked in vinegar. Cleopatra had herself rubbed daily with henna, olive oil, jasmine and other fragrant substances; the Empress Josephine used such huge quantities of musk that servants in her bedroom often fainted.

A third view was that of doctors who advised one to wash well and not to use any perfume because the "stinking crust interferes with the excretion of the impurities of which the skin is full."[286]

Historically, then, a shift in the appreciation of certain smells has occurred. For example, for us moderns the smell of valerian is a pungent, sweaty, "goaty" smell, and therefore not a particular favorite, but a few centuries ago this substance was used liberally to keep clothes "fresh" and possibly to mask all too unpleasant body odors. In the eighteenth and nineteenth centuries, the use of musk, amber and civet was generally discouraged: these "decaying substances" were supposed to have disastrous effects on mental health. It was believed that such substances irritate the nervous system and play into the hands of "feminist ideas." The use of flower smells—particularly rose, jasmine, orange blossom, mimosa, violet and hyacinth—was advised instead. If a woman covered herself with sweet smells, her spirit would no longer be sullied with animality.[287] Due to the admiration for ancient Greek and Roman culture, massage also became fashionable at that time, as did the taking of perfumed baths.

For their part, the Romans have left us a fine example of human tolerance for stench. The Romans washed white togas in old, stinking urine; the ammonia in the urine acted as a grease extractor and served as a bleaching agent. The Emperor Vespasian wanted to raise taxes on these laundries and on public urinals; the expression *pecunia non olet,* "money does not smell," derives from him.[288]

In many cultures perfumes and odors are associated with religious practices. We find countless passages about this in the Bible. Moses was given instructions for making an incense offering: "Take unto thee sweet spices, stacte, and onycha, and galbanum; these sweet spices with pure frankincense: of each there shall be a like weight: and thou shall make it a perfume, a confection after the art of the apothecary, tempered together, pure and holy: and thou shall beat some of it very small, and put of it before the testimony in the tabernacle of the congregation where I will meet with thee: it shall be unto you most holy" (Exodus 30: 34-37). Kings were anointed; Mary Magdalene washed Jesus's feet with myrrh, then dried them with her hair; the bride and bridegroom in the Song of Songs describe each other in terms of pleasant smells. One reason incense was burned in churches was to mask the smell of corpses. The use of incense was general and widespread, however. In ancient Egypt and in many other cultures, such as in Greece, incense sacrifices served to propitiate the gods and to cure people. Nero, for example, had tons of incense burned in order to enable the soul of Poppaea to find the right way to the afterlife.

Fragrances at the Present Time

Nowadays smells which, because of their appeal, once might have been considered "dangerous" can be used abundantly, because we have learned that a woman who smells nice is not automatically sexually available. So perfumes have a place in our culture apart from their ancient function of hiding odors. Once again: biologically, a perfume may contain pleasant olfactory signals, but because everyone who smells the perfume today realizes that it is artificial, a sexual response in the man is generally absent. That is, perfumes do not contain obvious information connected with sex.

This circumstance is the result of cultural evolution, which can put mechanisms which have arisen through biological evolution in different contexts, reversing or distorting their original meaning. This phenomenon is known even at the anatomical level: as a result of culture and upbringing, the "wiring" of our brains changes enormously in our early childhood.[289] From this perspective, perfumes are meant to create confusion: we smell something pleasant, but we are no longer meant to associate all kinds of behavior with the smell. It no longer refers to food, or to danger, and only in some cases—and certainly not without being supplemented by other sensory information—does it refer to a possible partner to be won. (A good example of these mixed signals is the perfume recently introduced onto the French market under the brand name Oui Non.)

The fact that animal pheromones such as musk are often ingredients in perfumes does not conflict with the view that the culturally determined significance of smells has come to dominate the biological function they may have had once. Such a pheromone might be intended to evoke a particular mood or feeling of sympathy among men, but that is not the same as the direct summoning of sexual behavior.[290] Moreover, a woman's nose is much more sensitive to musk (also called exaltolide) than a man's,[291] and perfumes often contain pheromone-like substances of a male nature, which women like and men precisely do not like. In short, perfumes are not primarily meant to make women sexually attractive to men (although perfumers sometimes think so), and as a rule women do not buy them for that reason.

Expensive substances are often incorporated in perfumes. Amber, derived from the intestines of the whale, costs nearly $60,000 a kilo. Precious civet is a secretion of a gland under the tail of the civet cat; in nature the smell has the function of deterring attackers. Musk in its natural form is derived from the male musk deer; the beaver produces a related substance. Because of the high cost of these substances, synthetic products (such as aldehydes) are often used nowadays.

Many perfumes even contain a slight smell of feces. That seems odder than it actually is. People do not have such an enormous revulsion to the smell of their own feces. Children often rub themselves with it, and adults often sit on the toilet longer than is necessary. The reason for this may be that feces are given a certain pheromone-like smell by glands situated close to the anus.[292] (Human feces also contain small concentrations of skatole and indole, which are found in jasmine.)

In the making of perfumes, the perfumer produces a mixture of these substances and countless others. A good perfume produces three types of smell in succession. First comes the "top note," when the most volatile ingredients are released—substances that generally smell fresh. Then follows the "heart" of the perfume—a full, warm smell. Finally there is an "after-fragrance," which surrounds the person for a long time.[293] The top note often consists of vegetable pheromones with which plants attract insects for pollination. The heart often contains animal pheromones.

The scent of a perfume depends somewhat on the person wearing it (as mentioned in Chapter 3). The temperature of the skin affects the speed of the evaporation of the fragrances, and substances found on the skin can react chemically with the perfume, creating unexpected olfactory effects. The perfume also interacts with the wearer's body odors, including those of the hair on one's head.

The perfume's scent seems to be linked to a certain extent with someone's personality structure as well. Treatises have been devoted to the optimum link between race, personality and perfume.[294] Extroverted people, for example, are supposed to be particularly attracted by fresh-smelling perfumes.

The Link with Emotions

Some researchers believe that in recent years the experience of smell has grown more and more refined because more and more fragrances are being produced, and that the range of our emotions and feelings has thereby grown, too.[295] A few people even go so far as to replace Descartes's adage *cogito ergo sum* (I think, therefore I am) with *olfacio ergo cogito* (I smell, therefore I think).[296] The substance of the claim is clear: more odors are supposed to evoke more emotions and feelings, and therefore lead to greater emotional development. The claim is difficult to investigate, for we cannot find out for sure whether our ancestors had more impoverished emotional lives *and* a different kind of sense of smell (it might be possible to investigate this through reports from earlier times about a fragrance we are familiar with but cannot smell).[297] It is at loggerheads with facts about the structure of our brains. Emotions and the sense of smell are mainly connected with the limbic system, with the cortex or the "neural chassis" and with the hypophysis. The rapid development and the intensive use of the neocortex have had consequences for our mental and cultural development and for the way emotions and feelings are expressed in language. The expression of emotions is completely different from the experience of emotions. Besides, current research in the field of intelligence suggests that socio-emotional and intellectual development are to a significant extent interdependent. The intellect may have produced a large number of new odors, but it does not follow from this that the limbic system has changed the way it functions.[298] Moreover, there are good reasons for assuming that this system has not developed structurally in man for tens of thousands of years.

It is worth noting that children often dislike perfume. That is sometimes said to be evidence that children are not yet aware of the aesthetic dimension of smells. It is more probable that the use of perfume by the mother is the cause of this aversion. The smell of perfume often means the parents are going out, not a pleasant event if it leads the child to fear being abandoned.

In general, there are links between emotions and all kinds of smells. Smells can reduce anxiety, make performance worse or better (mostly through conditioning), ease physical ailments and serve as aids in psychotherapy (see osmotherapy or aromatherapy in Chapter 8).[299] In a number of cases, phobias, depressions, sleep problems and addictions are claimed to be more easily treatable if certain smells are part of the remedy. Other smells are thought to have a relaxing effect—the smell of the sea, particularly. Tension of the facial muscles is said to reduce by about 20 percent in the presence of a "sea smell."[300]

The use of perfumes, too, may have to do with their supposed ability to reduce stress. If you ask a person why he or she uses perfume, the answer will probably be "I just like it," "It makes me feel fresh and well groomed" or "It gives me a lift" rather than "I do it for other people, I think it's important that other people should think I smell nice." That is, one's own sensory pleasure seems to play an important part in the decision to use perfumes.

The Use of Perfume and Context

The appraisal of a smell is highly dependent upon the context in which it is smelled. No one minds if you smell of sweat in the locker room, but an applicant for a job on the coaching staff would be advised not to sweat too much during the interview. A farmer wearing aftershave causes confusion; he is supposed to smell of manure. The car mechanic should be surrounded by the scents of rubber and oil and not of musk.

It does not matter if you stink provided the smell does not persist and its source is clearly something in the outside world—gasoline, oil, paint solvent. Pleasant smells, on the other hand, are often linked to one's personal qualities. Perhaps this phenomenon can be understood on the basis of the so-called fundamental attribution error: we have a tendency to attribute successes to ourselves and failures to factors originating outside us. When our vacation photographs turn out blurry, we blame it on the camera or the developer. If they're clear and sharp, we credit ourselves with a talent for photography. By analogy, if you smell nice due to a perfume, then it is because you are healthy and attractive; thus the perfume encourages us to act accordingly.

Given all this, it is astonishing that odors are used so little in order to guide our judgment of something or someone in a particular direction. It is known in ethnology that certimuli in animals often have pronounced effects on their behavior. The cuckoo makes use of its favorite host, the ruffed redstart, by laying a much larger egg in the nest, because the birds prefer brooding on the largest egg.[301]

In man, too, there are such "preferred stimuli." One well-known example is the *Kindchenschema*—that is, a pattern that evokes tenderness: a round face, large eyes, round cheeks, a chubby figure and the habit of making pleasant noises. Perhaps people prefer canaries to seagulls because the shape of the canary and the noises it makes fit better into the *Kindchenschema*. The canary provokes caring behavior in us, and as a result is treated nicely. The price that the animal pays for this is captivity, whereas seagulls have their freedom. Might perfumes also be such stimuli —that is, can perfumes make others feel affection for us, or are they limited to a kind of self-stimulation?

Commerce

It is far from easy to establish whether perfumes are pleasant or not. As we have observed, children often dislike perfumes, and the hedonic properties of odors are highly dependent on the social environment in which they are disseminated. "Intrinsically" pleasant smells scarcely exist. Anyone who tries to mask the smell of auto exhaust with Chanel No. 5 is sadly mistaken: the perfume will probably remind people of the daily misery of traffic jams.

Through advertising, the perfume manufacturer hopes to make the consumer believe he'll be able to emphasize his positive qualities by using the perfume. "Night Flight symbolizes the fervent desire of men for a new, individual identity. Night Flight, a new perspective in a man's life," read a flier distributed house to house by one pharmacy chain. The slogan was: "A boy's dream come true."

The pulling power of perfumes is determined more by marketing and various "foolish" intuitions than by solid research. Following on from what we have said about odor-driven behavior, we can state that the perfumes that women use have little to do with their conscious promotion of their attractiveness to men; that is fiction of the advertising industry. Even if perfumes have effects on one's sex life, that is not what motivates women to buy them; in fact, the point of the perfume may be to deter sexual approach.

It does not follow from this, however, that perfumes have no effect on other people. Experiments show that perfumes affect, for example, the ways in which job applicants are assessed.[302] A female student dressed in jeans and a T-shirt is regarded as attractive by her male colleagues when she uses a perfume, but the effect is lost when she dresses more formally, for then the lords of creation feel slightly uneasy, and the female student is more likely to be called "aloof" and "inaccessible." Other research indicates that men generally regard perfumed candidates (both women and men) as less suitable than unperfumed ones, less capable of doing the job and less appealing personally; women found perfumed applicants *more* suitable.

To explain these phenomena, the researchers put forward the following hypothesis: Men were distracted by the smell of the applicants. Perhaps they regarded the smell as an "insult" or as an attack on their capacity to make an objective judgment. In short, if you are a man, it may be useful to use fragrances in order to evoke a particular mood in women; if you are a woman, keep in mind that men prefer not to be confronted with either women or men who use perfumes, especially strong ones.

Clearly, the use of perfume plays a part in *impression management*, or the forming of a quick impression of a person. However, one has to be cautious: the influence of the fragrance becomes weaker if other tactics are used at the same time. Specifically, a woman involved with men can have too much of a good thing, too many influential stimuli. Perhaps that phenomenon is based on the fact that men are less able to process a complex construction of diverse sensory impressions in a "holistic" way.[303]

From a follow-up study on the application research, it emerged that when an applicant wearing perfume engaged in positive non-verbal communication—smiling, leaning in the direction of the interviewer—the questioners (especially men) were less able to remember what the applicant had said.[304] That is, the perfume undermined the effects of the body language. If you tend to make a good impression with body language, you should avoid perfume, but perfume may help if you are stiff when it comes to non-verbal communication.

Furthermore, many male university teachers know that it can be difficult to examine a seductively dressed, heavily perfumed female student orally. The examiners ask questions that are unclear and don't listen to the student's answers properly. As a result, the examination may become a succession of confusions and misunderstandings. A beautiful student would be advised to dress decorously and rather casually and to use at most a whiff of perfume. Possibly the questions posed to her will be more difficult (because the teacher is not distracted), but her answers will probably get through to him better.

To conclude: perfume does not have direct effects, certainly not as regards the opposite sex. The emotional and intellectual judgment of men tends to be generally undermined rather than improved by perfumes.

To formulate this in a negative way: men may be thrown into a state of mental confusion by perfumes. From an evolutionary perspective, that confusion may suit a woman living in a large group: in that way the monogamous bond necessary for bringing up the new generation has more chance of remaining intact. Any advances from men in the group often turn out to be in vain, and natural selection discourages a system with a large number of missed chances. Perhaps one can even say that odors give a woman better protection from undesirable approaches than knives and other weapons.

Some time ago—to give one example of how the marketplace has responded to such thinking—a vial was put on the market for women (at least they are the target group) to use in defending themselves against attackers. The vial is fastened to the bra with a clip, and is meant to be broken in the event of danger; a few seconds later a disgusting smell, a little like burning rubber, is given off, which makes the attacker vomit (it makes the woman vomit as well).[305]

Summing up, again, we can say that women often use perfumes because they like them, and not primarily because they want to please men. (In the words of an advertising brochure: "Escada Light is a perfect supplement for those moments in the day when you want to enjoy a sensual, feminine, luxurious fragrance more intensely.") A visit to the perfume department in a department store supports this line of thought. Usually women also buy a perfume for their partners, or often use "male" fragrances themselves because they find them more attractive.

In short, perfumes are not artificial pheromones. Women mainly *like* perfumes; but if a man wants to enhance his appearance, scents can help him.

Olfactory Passports and Animal Performance

In the animal kingdom, pheromones elicit certain behavior, whether or not in a compulsive way. With mankind, however, the situation is more complicated. If each of us has a personal aroma or body odor—an "olfactory passport"—the recognition and appreciation of it is not dependent on a particular substance (that is, a pheromone present in everyone). What matters in the body odor is the sum of all the odors given off by the person. A person's olfactory passport is connected with race and upbringing, among other things. The question is: How can an olfactory organ recognize another person from his or her aroma or body odor? And if it can, why? What is the function of that behavior?

We are rarely aware of our own body odor, unless it suddenly changes. One reason for this is that we are habituated to it; and there are indications that we are loath to be intimate with people whose aromas contrast strongly with our own, and drawn instead to people who "fit in with" our own olfactory passport.

The characteristics of body odor are, as has been said, closely connected with factors such as eating habits, hygiene and living conditions, values seen in the aggregate as the *chemosphere*. During wars, warring parties even tried to recognize each other on the basis of "wafting" body odors.[306] There are indications that the sweat of anxious people (and animals) takes on a special smell. Physical (and possibly genetic) factors like the distribution and operation of the sweat glands leave their mark on the olfactory passport as well. And it has been shown that there are great cultural differences in the strength of the body odor, particularly the armpit sweat, whose intensity is largely determined by the number of sweat glands. Blacks and Koreans represent extremes; perhaps this is why some Koreans and other Asians find blacks' body odor to be strong and unpleasant.[307]

That a person's hereditary background helps to determine his or her personal odor has been established in a research project in which four dogs with sufficient retrieval experience tried to distinguish human twins from each other from their smells.[308] Both identical and non-identical twins (fifty pairs in all) wore a T-shirt for twenty-four hours; then the shirts were put into plastic bags. Each dog was allowed to sniff a T-shirt for fifteen seconds; afterward—with the dog no longer present—the shirt was put next to the shirt worn by the other twin. Subsequently the dog had to retrieve the shirt on command.

The results of the experiment were striking. On average the dogs were able to distinguish the T-shirts of the genetically different twins from each other, and identified over 80 percent of the T-shirts of the genetically identical twins. Some pairs of both kinds of twins had different living conditions, however, and this caused the dogs quite often to hesitate in making their choice. The dogs could *not* distinguish the T-shirts worn by identical twins who had the same living conditions and ate the same food. (As a control, the dogs were prompted to smell shirts that had not been worn. They retrieved these shirts at random.) The results may be ascribed to differences in the body odors of the twins (and not to any other smells in the house where they lived); the conclusion is that there is a hereditary factor involved in body odor. A dog's sense of smell is therefore sufficiently developed to be able to distinguish people on the basis of their body odor, provided the genetic structure and/or the living environment of one person differs from that of the other.

Recognizing Each Other's Body Odor

Can human beings identify each other (and themselves) on the basis of their smells? A related experiment attempted to answer this question. A hundred people were asked to "fetch" their own T-shirt. They had worn the shirt for twenty-four hours, without using any soap, deodorant or perfume,[309] and deviating as little as possible from their normal patterns of life and eating habits. The shirts were put into bags; after a number of days, the people had to try to fish out their own shirts from a collection of ten bags containing identical shirts belonging to themselves and nine other people. Three-quarters of the people were able to identify their own shirt. Among those who failed, a number were heavy smokers, people younger than twenty and menstruating women; a proportionately large number of those who failed were men. In a similar study, only 30 percent of the people had been able to retrieve their own T-shirt, but in that study they were given much less time to make their choice.[310] If you give people the opportunity to get a good whiff, then they will smell much better.

These experiments suggest that we are able to recognize our own olfactory passport, provided the olfactory organ is given sufficient time and has gained enough experience in learning to distinguish subtle differences in smell, and provided the sense of smell has not suffered greatly from tobacco smoke. In addition, women have this capacity rather more markedly than men, except during menstruation. In that period their sensitivity to smells declines sharply, perhaps due to changes in the concentration of various hormones, such as luteinizing hormone (LH), follicle-stimulating hormone (FSH) and progesterone.[311]

Having established that we can recognize our own smell, the next question is an obvious one: Do we also achieve reasonable results with other people's smell? We will not summarize all the facts described here, but will concentrate on what is known about the olfactory bond between mother and child and between members of families.

Parents and Children

Various studies have shown that mothers have little difficulty in recognizing their infants on the basis of the smell they give off.[312] Twenty mothers were asked to smell the swaddling clothes that had been wrapped around the babies immediately after birth and left on them for twenty-four hours. Eighty percent of mothers were able to identify their own child's blanket. It made no difference whether the newborn child had been born in a normal way or by caesarean section. Nor did it matter whether the child was a boy or a girl, whether the mother had given birth before or whether the mother nursed the child from the breast or from a bottle. It did matter, however, that the test was taken a number of days after the birth, or shortly before mother and child were discharged from the hospital. The mother had had ample opportunity to smell her baby's smell, making recognition easier.

Another experiment investigated whether mothers who had had little contact with their child were able to recognize the child's swaddling clothes on the basis of smell. Seventeen mothers who had given birth through caesarean section were asked to identify the clothes twenty-four hours after birth. This experiment was significantly different from the previous one, in that in a birth through caesarean section there is scarcely any contact between mother and child early on because the mother is drowsy or nauseous from the anesthetic, and so has little opportunity to get to know her baby's smell. In any case, three-quarters of these mothers were able to produce the correct cloth, a significant result. We do not know how the process of recognition of smell, between mother and child operates: perhaps the imprinting happens very quickly.

Other researchers had come to similar conclusions, and had reported a remarkable incidental phenomenon: on the fifth and sixth days after the birth of the child there was a clear decline in the mother's olfactory recognition.[313] This might be connected with the physiological changes both in the mother and in the child. The infant acquires an increasingly personal smell, which is much less like that of amniotic fluid, whereas the mother might develop a temporarily inferior sensitivity to smell because of changes in her hormonal levels (just as during menstruation).

Of course, it has also been investigated whether the newborn child can recognize its mother through smell. In an experiment, gauze bandage was put over the body zones important in feeding—the mother's breasts, neck, cheeks and shoulders. Later, one of the bandages was hung to one side of the child's head in the crib, with a bandage from a strange mother on the other side. The movements of the infants were filmed. A frame-by-frame analysis of the material showed that the child's face and arm were directed much more often to the side of its own mother's bandage than to the strange mother's side.[314] If only a bandage from its own mother was hung up, moreover, the child moved much less often than when a bandage from another mother or a non-impregnated piece of gauze was hanging in the crib—that is, the child was calmer. On the basis of these facts we can reasonably say that, at least initially, there is a link between the smell of mother and child, and that the smell of the mother is recognized by the child.

From a related experiment, it appears that the smell of the father is not more appreciated by the baby than the smell of a strange man.[315] "Genetic recognizability" and "genetic affinity" do not mean very much in this context: the most important thing is the *contact* experienced with the mother. Breast feeding is important: bottle-fed babies show scarcely any preference for their mother compared with any other woman. It also follows from these facts that babies will like their father's smell more, the more he concerns himself with the baby.

Are outsiders able to use their sense of smell to determine which child belongs to which mother?[316] To answer this question, a large number of T-shirts were ordered. Mother and child had to wear the garments, observing the previously mentioned rules. A total of twenty-eight test subjects, who were not related to or familiar with mother and child, smelled the T-shirt worn by the baby. Subsequently they had to try to retrieve the T-shirt worn by the mother from a group of four. Approximately half the people succeeded in doing this (the random expectation is one-quarter). This does not imply that the smell of the mother and the child were judged to be identical: it is possible that the test subjects simply regarded the smell of the mother as more similar to that of the baby than were the smells of other mothers. As would be expected, people who are related to mother and child perform equally well or even better in this respect. Other members of the family—such as fathers, aunts and grandmothers—were asked to identify a newborn child via sheets without their being any appreciable previous contact;[317] 26 of the 30 fathers were able to do this, 15 of the 20 aunts and 15 of 20 grandmothers. It emerged from other studies that fathers are *not* able to recognize their child on the basis of smell, but in those experiments the selection procedure had been made considerably more difficult.[318] Another experiment involved married couples wearing the T-shirts. Only 10 of 28 test subjects were able to combine two shirts in the correct way, a result no different from random selection.

It seems therefore the olfactory bond between the mother and the child is somewhat stronger than that between grown-ups who have a permanent relationship, which is also the case with animals (Chapter 1). Moreover, it follows that similar surroundings or living habits cannot make people develop the same body odor: probably each person's chemical signature is also partly determined by his hereditary background.

To summarize: Members of nuclear and extended families can recognize each other's olfactory signature to a certain extent, as can brothers and sisters who have been separated for some time (longer than a month). Nevertheless, we must be cautious in making sweeping statements on the degree to which similarities in smell are based on genetic relationship or on environmental influences. Possibly brothers and sisters recognize each other's smells even after a period of separation because at an earlier stage they had a familiar and intense bond.

Smell and Parental Care

We saw in the discussion of pheromones that these substances are generally perceived unconsciously, and that their operation is far from unambiguous or direct. The function of sex pheromones is unclear, and not infrequently the facts lend themselves to differing interpretations. We must not conclude, however, that a person's body odor plays no significant role. The personal aroma consists of countless volatile substances that can change in concentration and composition; while no single component is decisive, the impression made by the whole can be of great importance.

It is certain, in any case, that smells play a significant role in the upbringing of children and animals (as seen in Chapter 1). Another example from the animal kingdom: it has been shown in rats that young whose olfactory bulbi or olfactory organs are damaged feed less, and even starve to death.[319] It is suspected that the smell of the mother during suckling causes the production of endorphins in the brain of the young; by conditioning the young to a feeling of pleasure, these odors may ensure a stronger bond between it and the mother. The smells may affect the mother, too, adding pleasure to the child's sucking, which is by no means painless. In a more general sense, odors seem to promote certain reactions (possibly again through the production of endorphins), for parts of the brain involved directly in smell are strikingly rich in receptors sensitive to these endorphins.[320]

For the newborn human infant, too, smells reinforce the mechanisms that shape and maintain bonding and dependence. This process can operate in various ways.[321] Small children generally learn to recognize and attach a meaning to a smell—often a pleasant one—very quickly; often the child needs help and will focus on smells that it comes into contact with most. (Indeed, the child may prefer an arbitrary smell that may not originate in the human body to another, unknown smell, provided the child is exposed to it for an extended period.[322]) Smells, of course, also enable the infant to recognize its own environment; both children and young animals prefer contact with their own mother, even if there has previously been little contact.[323]

Smells, in addition to influencing children's behavior, affect their bodily functions. Familiar smells calm a crying child and pacify him. Generally, the mother's smell reduces a child's anxiety, as seen in the way toddlers who are separated from their mothers become attached to pillowcases, items of their mother's clothing and suchlike—provided that the objects retain the mother's smell.

In short, smells confirm and perpetuate the bond between people. The *quality* of the smells is more or less unimportant. One can get used to almost anything. Few people believe that their partner stinks (so long as the relationship is good), or that their parents, brothers, sisters and friends smell unpleasant. Even though these people may smell unpleasant according to "objective" criteria, they give us attention, love and care, factors that through conditioning can lend positive associations to a virtually arbitrary body smell.

That smell is important for the connection between parent and child, and for those living in families, also emerged from research with animals other than mammals. Reptiles must make do without an olfactory cortex (paleocortex) and it may be for this reason that they have little interest in their offspring (except for crocodiles and lizards).[324] Birds probably do not bond on the basis of smells either; they generally have a poor sense of smell and follow the first object that moves when they emerge from the egg.

Breath Smells of Men and Women

What about the smell of the breath of men and women? Many men use breath fresheners, and that this phenomenon may have a deeper meaning than those seen in the movies can be deduced from research conducted into the smell of human breath, and more specifically into its hedonic quality.[325]

Men and women were recruited from the dental faculty of a university to investigate whether the smell of a person's breath says anything about the sex of the person. The donors blew into a glass tube that issued into a funnel; the smell was inhaled by panel members who were on the other side of a wooden partition. The results confirmed that women on average smell more acutely than men. Women panelists identified the sex of 90 percent of men by their breath, and 80 percent of the women. The male members of the panel did not do badly; they identified the sex of 65 percent of the donors. Notably, women found the men's breath smell stronger and less pleasant than other men did. Because men smell less acutely, they may have more trouble in smelling breath smells well, and be less bothered by foul breath. Similar experiments using armpit sweat and the sweat from the palms of the hands produced similar results: women and men were able to establish the sex of the donor very well and reasonably well, respectively.[326]

An amusing phenomenon: when a woman had an unpleasant breath smell, the female members of the panel often thought she was a man. In other words, men and women do not in the first instance distinguish between the sexes; they associate a stronger and a more unpleasant breath smell with a man, as they do with body odor generally. On the one hand, this could suggest that men should avoid breath fresheners, which mask a man's "male smell"—and make him less "manly"; on the other hand, men might wish to sweeten their foul breath. Remember the *aura seminalis* of the man, and the idea that women are supposed to smell of milk.

Chapter 8

Olfactory Disorders

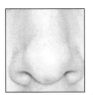**F**ew structural faults or innate defects are found in the olfactory apparatus, which is a quite simple organ compared, for example, with the complicated eye, which can be affected by many problems: refraction errors (which can be remedied with lenses), clouding of the cornea, cataracts, increased pressure (glaucoma), disintegration of the vitreous humor, countless ailments of the retina, detachment of the retina, degeneration of the fovea (the pit-shaped area of the retina with which we see in sharpest focus), etc. And while many people are born blind or deaf, an innate inability to smell is rare. Albinos are an exception to this; a particular genetic defect may result in an absence of odor-binding proteins (see Chapter 2). Perhaps the simplicity of the olfactory organ is also one of the reasons why there are no specialized smell doctors. First a few general observations.

Cultural Evolution, Life Expectancy, Prejudices

Strictly speaking, our biological life expectancy is not known. That is because, in contrast to animals, humans have two forms of evolution: biological and cultural. By virtue of cultural evolution we create a large part of our environment ourselves: clothes, houses, art, science, technology, transportation. Animals are able to manipulate their environment far less than we do, though to a certain extent the constructions of termites and bees are exceptions.

Cultural evolution also helps determine life expectancy. Due to "progress," a fair number of people have achieved a relatively good existence; yet enormous numbers of people scarcely profit from progress. In developing countries, the average human being lives for only forty years, partly because of poor nutrition, high infant mortality and poor hygiene. The average ancient Greek lived to be thirty-five, as did Western Europeans in the Middle Ages, while the present life expectancy at birth in the United States is 72 years for men and 79 years for women. This difference is to a large extent unexplained, although more men than women die through accidents and occupational illnesses.

In contrast to what is generally claimed, the markedly increased life expectancy is only to a small extent due to medicine. Obviously, postnatal care, the pasteurizing of milk, water purification and immunization against disease have lengthened our lives.[327] It is estimated that medical science in the narrower sense has added only about three years to life expectancy over the last century, and that gain is mainly in "qualitatively unhealthy" additional years of old age.[328] And in many areas—such as cancer, rheumatism, asthma—for decades there has been no substantial progress in terms of the chances of recovery.[329]

On the other hand, the positive influence of good nutrition on health and life expectancy is still underestimated. For example, it is probable that a reasonable consumption of vitamin C increases the life expectancy of men by no less than six years and that of women by one year, and there are estimates that the onset of a third of all cancers could be delayed or even prevented through better nutrition.[330]

Etiology is the medical specialization that maps the causes of disease. It is subject to increasing criticism, even among etiologists themselves. In the Western tradition, illnesses are seldom regarded as results of a large number of processes and factors. Medical theory and practice are still dominated by monocausal thinking, reductionism, and relatively simple determinism: illnesses are supposed to be generally traceable to one primary cause, and in principle can be dispelled through a single remedy.

This train of thought issues from the mechanized view of the world that emerged in the Enlightenment, which interpreted everything that happened in reality as a mechanical process. Just as in a clock one cogwheel was set in motion by another, so everything had in principle a primary cause, it was thought (as today, for example, in the case of AIDS and the HIV virus: anyone maintaining that there may be more factors involved in AIDS is branded as an idiot[331]). This view also understands man as directed primarily by *reason* and not by emotions, the body or by the senses, such as smell.

In the natural sciences particularly, this way of thinking has led to great successes, but not all processes connected with sickness and health can be assimilated to it. (For example, psychosomatic factors play a part in no less than two-thirds of all medical consultations.) Yet medicine tends to follow general views of human beings and the world for a long time, even if a particular approach has proved unfruitful. As far as smell is concerned, the consequence is that there has been little research in the field of diagnostics and treatment of olfactory disorders: this sense enjoys very little prestige in medicine.

Handicapped?

That is a shame, because our sense of smell is not in good shape. A decline in or even complete loss of the ability to smell is quite a common disorder. People with such disorders are generally not regarded as handicapped, although such defects can have unpleasant and even dangerous consequences. The afflicted person does not realize it when meat is spoiled, food is burning or a gas leak has started in the basement. Without smell much of life loses its quality, not only in the culinary field but also in an emotional and sexual respect—you must be able to *smell* your partner.

Those changes in the emotional field have to do with the fact

that the olfactory nerves are particularly connected to the old limbic system, the part of the brain that is of great importance for
emotions and feelings. An olfactory disorder is consequently often
followed by depression, perhaps because smells are an important
"input" of the limbic system and of the right hemisphere of the
brain. (The reverse—that depression is supposed to lead to the
loss of smell—can scarcely be supported by argument; in addition
innate anosmia is not often linked to an increased likelihood of
the development of depression.)

When the sense of smell is seriously weakened, the episodic
memory may function less efficiently as well, since the sense of
smell activates memories (Chapter 5). However, olfactory problems are not always independent phenomena: often a reduced capacity for smell is linked to some physical or mental ailment.[332]
Finally there is a possibility of a changed, even a significantly
better-functioning olfactory sense.

A person who lost his sense of smell was amazed by how much
he lost.[333] "Sense of smell," he said. "I never gave it a thought.
You don't normally give it a thought. But when I lost it—it was
like being struck blind. . . . You *smell* people, you *smell* the city,
you *smell* the spring—maybe not consciously, but as a rich unconscious background to everything else. My world was suddenly
radically poorer."

Innate Defects

Only a small portion of the population suffers from innate anosmia
or a general inability to smell. But many people have innate limited
anosmias—that is, they cannot smell certain odors. People so afflicted often do not realize it; like color blindness, it can remain
unnoticed for a long time, only to emerge through a test during
a medical examination. Specific "olfactory blindness" may be
caused by the absence of certain odorant-binding proteins in the
olfactory epithelium (see Chapter 2).[334]

A greater number of people suffer from limited anosmia. For
example, 10 percent of people are anosmic for prussic acid, and
almost half for androstenone.[335] However, experiments in this field

take no account of the possibility that an unconsciously perceived smell may have been noticed by the olfactory organ and affect behavior and mood even so.

This phenomenon can be compared with *blind sight*. People afflicted with blind sight (a result of an injury to the optical cortex in the brain) cannot see but remain aware of obstacles, which they perceive at an unconscious level. A similar phenomenon exists with the sense of touch (*blind touch*): patients are able to adapt their hand to the form of an object that they do not consciously feel. Analogously we might speak of *blind smell*: we often react to smells even though we cannot smell them consciously. You could even say that this phenomenon is characteristic of smell in general; it would appear that for a large part of the day we do not smell anything.[336] Again, this is not surprising. In evolutionary terms, the "old" parts of the brain predominate in the perception of smells; these have relatively indirect connections with the neo-cortex (and hence with language ability and self-consciousness) and more direct connections with the many "automatic pilots" that guide our actions. It is obvious, however, that one can speak of *blind smell* only if the olfactory organ itself is not anosmic for the relevant substances (just as the eye is not blind in the case of *blind sight*).

One of the most common causes of innate anosmia is Kallman's syndrome, a hormonal affliction that occurs mainly in men.[337] The ailment is caused by a recessive gene not resting on a sex chromosome. In boys the illness is characterized by a retarded development of the penis and testicles in puberty; they remain hairless. Afflicted girls have slim hips, small breasts and little pubic hair, and do not menstruate. Yet these people are not eunuchs. What they lack are certain "stimulants," probably because the gene "in its dominant form" produces too little of a certain protein essential for the manufacture of the relevant hormones. A moderate dose of sex hormones may *perhaps* prevent too great a retardation of development in puberty.[338]

Men with Kallman's syndrome have little testosterone in their blood (0.2 to 0.3 nanogram per milliliter, as opposed to 3 to 8 nanograms per milliliter in normal men).[339] A low concentration of this hormone can mean that the sense of smell scarcely develops. Remarkably enough, the olfactory *organ* is generally in order in these people, as are the nerve connections with the brain. If we look at the rhinencephalon of patients with these symptoms, however, we are struck by the fact that a particular twist in the olfactory system is missing, and the hypothalamus also has a defective structure.[340] It looks as though certain parts of the brain have not fully matured, and this stunted growth also affects sexual development. The administering of hormones may help to preserve some of the ability to smell, but more research is needed.

Acquired Disorders

The sense of smell can be afflicted with the following acquired disorders, called olfactory dysfunctions:

- *General anosmia:* the inability to smell any odor.
- *Limited anosmia:* the inability to smell certain odors.
- *Hyposmia:* a reduced capacity to smell all odors.
- *Hyperosmia:* oversensitivity to some or all odors.
- *Dysosmia:* a smell disorder characterized by constantly changing, random smell sensations.
- *Fantosmia:* a form of dysosmia in which mainly unpleasant odors are smelled, without the ability to identify substances in the surroundings responsible for these sensations—a kind of olfactory hallucination, that is.
- *Parosmia:* a form of dysosmia in which the characteristics of an odor change regularly.
- *Kakosmia:* a kind of parosmia in which one's appreciation of odors changes radically, so that odors once found pleasant now seem to stink. With this affliction even eating can become difficult.
- *Agnosia:* the inability to name odors and distinguish them, although the sense of smell is otherwise normal. The person with this affliction mentions a sensation, but cannot name or interpret it.

In the United States millions of people suffer from one or more of these ailments; unfortunately, there is a lack of reliable recent data about the degree to which olfactory disorders occur in other countries and about their distribution over various occupational groups. Epidemiological research is still in its infancy, and many inventories were created in an inadequate way.[341] The experts themselves are not to blame: thorough research is costly and difficult to undertake without the support of medical services and government aid.

We also see that the importance of the sense of smell for the quality of life is underestimated. People who have problems with their sense of sight or hearing can often do something about it by consulting a specialist. The audiologist gives us a hearing aid, the optician or optometrist fits us with a pair of glasses or contact lenses. In the field of smell disorders, however, there are virtually no experts. The manner in which ear, nose and throat doctors or neurologists investigate a smell disorder (let alone treat it) is not worthy of the name of medicine. Often only about three odors are used to determine the loss of smell. Moreover, the patient is often asked to *name* the substances. That is not a very sensible method: we know that smells particularly have effective meanings, which generally are not easy to express in language, and that being *able* to smell and/or recognize a smell is very different from naming it. These doctors also sometimes use substances that the patient is meant to perceive through stimulation of the trigeminal nerve, which has nothing to do with the sense of smell properly.

A number of years ago a smell test was devised—the UPSIT: University of Pennsylvania Smell Identification Test.[342] It turned out that approximately 1 percent of the population was able to identify less than half the forty odors used in this test via multiple-choice questions. Such data are used to assess the degree to which a person is anosmic. The borderline for hyposmia is at a point where someone registers a score exceeded by at least 90 percent of people of the same age: meaning that 90 percent smell better than the subject. It is clear that anosmia and hyposmia are fairly arbitrary categories.[343] It does not follow, though, that people who score low in the test constantly suffer from olfactory disorders: the sense of smell is often seriously affected by a cold or by inflammation of the mucous membrane. Usually the patient recovers, although in some cases that may take months. The UPSIT test, then, is only a snapshot, and is not suitable for mapping "the" ability to smell of "the" population.

Only a few people have specialized in diagnosing olfactory disorders.[344] These specialists use large numbers of odors in various concentrations. In order to be able to assess the patient's degree of loss of smell, the smell-identification test was first administered to normal people, so that there is comparative material available.

Causes and Treatment

The causes of olfactory disorders can be divided into three groups: virus infections, including ordinary colds; pathological processes in the nasal cavities, such as inflammation of the mucous membrane, jaw, or sinuses; and injuries or traumas such as a fall or a blow to the head. Traumatic damage to the olfactory organ occurs much more often in men than in women: generally speaking, men are more likely to have traffic accidents or accidents at work.

Such injuries occur in the following ways: The brain more or less "swims" in the skull, surrounded by a liquid, the *liquor cerebrospinalis*. When there is a hard blow to the head the brain twists somewhat, particularly if the blow comes from the side. The olfactory nerves "scrape" across the rough base of the skull, and the loss of smell results. Another Achilles' heel in the system involves the nerve fibers of the sensory cells, which make contact with the rhinencephalon through perforations in the ethmoid bone. If there is a heavy shock or collision (for example, when the head is thrown forward, which happens quite often in traffic accidents), the nerve fibers may be severed by the edges of the ethmoid bone. Initially nothing seems to be wrong, until the victim starts eating in the evening. He may still be able to perceive some smells, but he soon realizes that something is wrong. If all connections are severed, then the prognosis is bad. Because no more olfactory information comes in, the nerve cells in the rhinencephalon eventually die off, like unused muscles.[345] The olfactory organ itself sometimes remains intact, and often the sensory cells are able to make new connections with the brain, so that there may be some degree of recovery after a number of months. However, this improvement, which happens not infrequently after such a trauma, is often linked with fantosmia and kakosmia, unpleasant phenomena akin to the visual hallucinations that often accompany migraines.

Anosmia that occurs as a result of a concussion or a blow to the head often leads to changes in the victim's eating behavior, because smell and taste cooperate closely. The chance of eating disorders is greater still if *hypogeusia*, or a decline in taste, strikes as well. That phenomenon can appear when there is an injury to the seventh brain nerve, the *nervus facialis*. This nerve is responsible for movements in the face; one of its branches (the *chorda tympani*) also plays a part in taste.[346]

In the case of anorexia nervosa, too, a smell or taste disorder may have aggravated the problem. Such a disorder can sometimes contribute to the emergence of bulimia, possibly because the patient is desperately trying to stimulate her sense of smell and taste.[347]

In the United States, the consensus of experts working from research performed in the late 1970s was that nearly 2 million citizens had a smell disorder of some kind, and more recently the National Institute on Deafness and Other Communication Disorders has estimated that more than 200,000 Americans visit a doctor for a smell or taste disorder each year. Here, as in Europe, the causes of olfactory disorders are various. Some people are born with a smell disorder; for others, the loss of smell can be traced back to concussions or other injuries, to upper respiratory infections, or to viral infections. Among the complications alluded to are inflammations of the mucous membrane (rhinitis), which is often the result of an allergy, and infections of the jaw and sinuses. A striking and unexplained fact is that many more men than women are affected by loss of smell after concussions, while women more often develop a certain degree of hyposmia after a viral infection.

The prognosis in the loss of smell is not always unfavorable: one-third to one half of people who have developed an olfactory disorder as a result of a trauma experience a spontaneous recovery within one year. When the problem is caused by viral infections, victims recover similarly but their recovery is generally less pronounced and it takes place more slowly than in accident victims. Patients whose smell problems were caused by pathology in the nasal cavities have reasonable prospects.

The treatment of olfactory disorders is difficult. Therapy is possible, particularly if the cause of the defect lies in the nasal cavities, in which case administering adrenal hormones (such as prednisone) sometimes helps. High and long-term dosages of those substances, however, produce serious side effects, such as impaired functioning of the adrenal gland, obesity in the upper body, cataracts, thinning of the skin, loss of bone mass and depression. These hormones often have only a temporary effect: when the patient stops taking them, he loses his sense of smell again. Cleaning and operating on the nasal cavities may also help in some cases.

Over the years, countless other medicines have been administered for olfactory disorders, such as zinc compounds and even strychnine, but there is no reason to assume that those substances help. It is sometimes argued that zinc sulphate ($ZnSO_4$) aids the recovery of the sense of smell to some extent; the assumption is that poor nutrition has caused a shortage of trace elements essential for smell, which are compensated for by zinc sulphate (sometimes copper sulphate). A double-blind study, however, registered no striking improvement of this sort.[348] Finally, the drip feeding of cocaine is supposed to have reduced some patients' problems with parosmia—but this does not mean that their sense of smell improved.

Summarizing, we can say that olfactory disorders are as troublesome as they are difficult to treat. A good diagnosis is important because then the problem (particularly when it is in the nasal cavities) can be treated with therapy.

Smell and Disease

Both our physical and our mental condition affect the operation of the senses and parts of the brain which are connected with it. An attack of migraine (particularly *migraine ophtalmique*) is often linked with visual hallucinations in the form of flashes of light and "serrations," indicating that there is a shortage of blood supply to the visual system in the brain. In such circumstances there is no point in reading or writing a book, even if one wants to. Another remarkable phenomenon is *palinopsia*, by which the brain, when the retina is damaged, tries to complete the picture of the outside world via a kind of hallucination.

A less dramatic phenomenon, also connected with general physical condition, is the experience that the quality of the smell of roasting is significantly less marked after a full meal than before. The intensity of smells also appears to decline sharply under those circumstances (which is partly a result of adaptation). This variation in smell sensation and intensity as a product of one's general physiological condition, again, is called alliesthesia. The smell of lemonade syrup is pleasant to someone who is hungry, less so to the person who has just eaten sugary foods.[349] So there is a certain balance or link between the intensity and the appreciation of a smell and the general condition of the person.

With illnesses such phenomena can take on troublesome forms. Many illnesses, syndromes and psychoses have destructive effects on the capacity to smell.[350] A psychosis may be accompanied by a sudden change in the appreciation of smell: things that smelled pleasant yesterday stink today. Sometimes chronic problems with smell can be traced back to changes—side effects of medication—in the state of the olfactory epithelium and of the rhinencephalon. The use of certain antidepressants, for example, inhibit the creation of new sensory cells in the olfactory epithelium (Chapter 2). With long-term use of such a substance the number of sensory cells declines. This side effect is not usually mentioned, though loss of smell can cause or aggravate depression.[351] Radiotherapy (for cancer) can also have a devastating effect on the sense of smell.

Often the loss of smell relates to disorders connected with the nasal cavity, in which, for example, the stream of air across the olfactory epithelium is blocked. The cause of this can be anything from a common cold to a malignant tumor in a nasal cavity which has spread in the direction of the olfactory organ. Sometimes careless surgery, as in the removal of nasal polyps, causes damage and loss of smell. Viral infections such as herpes and hepatitis can have harmful effects on smell, as can disruptions and changes in the hormonal balance: during the menstrual cycle women show a great variation in their sensitivity to many odors. Illnesses connected with a reduced production of sex hormones often result in a reduction in the capacity to smell; and finally, diabetes leads in a number of cases to a less efficient functioning of the olfactory organ.

There are also some very strange associated phenomena. Illnesses and disorders like epilepsy often go hand in hand with hyperosmia (oversensitivity to smells). Epileptic fits are frequently heralded by an olfactory hallucination, and such attacks can sometimes even be triggered by smells. Multiple sclerosis quite often leads to hyposmia, as do Parkinson's disease and other syndromes connected with dementia, such as Alzheimer's disease, Korsakoff's psychosis and Huntington's chorea. Patients who complain about constantly changing or strange smells but who are otherwise very much alert may have developed one of these disorders in a latent form.

With smell and illness in general, the doctor should use his nose more often in making diagnoses.[352] Sometimes illness has an aroma; various ailments are even characterized by an unmistakable smell. Illnesses like lung cancer, stomach cancer, yellow fever, typhus, measles, diphtheria and diabetes are linked to a specific breath and body odor; in the case of diabetes, the breath may smell of acetone or be "sickly sweet"; poor kidney function often leads to a fishy smell, and the smell of garlic sometimes indicates poisoning.[353] Inappropriate prudery often inhibits doctors from paying attention to the smell a person gives off through his bodily orifices (including the pores), although the smell may confirm or disprove a diagnosis.[354] Moreover, the doctor rarely takes into account the possible diagnostic significance of a reduced or changed sense of smell when he is looking for the cause of pathological phenomena: a disorder of smell may be a symptom of, for example, a brain tumor or the onset of dementia.

Of course, we have to be careful not to link a loss of the capacity for smell directly with serious illnesses, because even a simple cold can have serious effects on the sense of smell. But if the complaints are chronic, a smell test can have a useful diagnostic function. Such a test is inexpensive and the patient can often administer it himself (the UPSIT test is one; the University of Utrecht in the Netherlands has developed another, the Smell Identification Test Utrecht, or GITU).[355]

As we saw in Chapter 1, smell historically has played an important part in medicine: it was thought that bodily smells revealed the composition and quality of the vital juices.[356] Hippocrates spoke of "the smell of health," and the "sickly smell," which allegedly meant that "sour" was replaced by "alkaline." In addition, all kinds of diseases—so said the doctors in the past— have specific odors. "Doctors know the smell of gangrene and cancer virus and bone degeneration," says Corbin. Wards in hospitals were also distinguished on the basis of their smells. "Where there are children, the smell is sour and stinks; where women are lying, sweet and rotting; in the male wards, there is a strong smell, which stinks but is much less repellent." Finally, illnesses were often connected to processes of decay, which were accordingly investigated thoroughly. A thesis of 1760 contains a "sequence" of the smell of cadavers: sickening, sour, pungently repellent, spicy and finally the smell of amber. The author of the dissertation concludes with a recommendation: "This should encourage doctors to identify the smells of sick people with more precision." These views on the link between smell and sickness led ordinary people to pay close attention to the smells of burping, belching, flatulence, urine and feces.

Hormonal Disorders

Abnormal hormone levels can have both reinforcing and destructive effects on the sense of smell. A tumor of the hypophysis can lead women to produce more estrogen, so that the sense of smell improves considerably. Addison's disease, which involves a poorly operating adrenal gland, also leads to hyperosmia. In these patients, the threshold value for many odors is frequently 10,000 times as low as in healthy people. These people can smell sugar, urea and highly diluted hydrochloric acid, substances that normally can only be tasted.[357] In Addison's disease the production of glucocorticoids by the adrenal gland falls sharply. When patients who take large quantities of these hormones (as treatments for asthma and rheumatism) suddenly stop taking them, a "crisis of Addison" is caused, with comparable results. Glucocorticoids, like sex hormones, are steroids, but these "stress hormones" have an important function in converting fat and protein into carbohydrates. Obviously they are of great importance to the synaptic transfer of nerve impulses connected with smell. They exert an inhibiting effect; when there is a shortage of glucocorticoids, administering these hormones (in the form of prednisone) returns the sense of smell to normal.

Dementia

Dementia is characterized by the sudden failure of higher brain functions. This form of decay may have all kinds of causes, such as a series of minor heart attacks, hemorrhages and of course the mysterious Alzheimer's disease.[358] It is striking that systems in the brain formed at an early stage in evolution generally suffer less from such degeneration phenomena—even illnesses and tumors. For example, the brain stem, which helps to control such bodily functions as breathing and heartbeat, is strong and tough and can survive for a relatively long time without oxygen.

In discussions of dementia the sense of smell is generally not mentioned. The rhinencephalon belongs to the phylogenetically old structures, which are somewhat less prone to wear and tear and decay. Recently, however, it came to light that a "limited" degeneration in those systems is an important step in the development of dementia.[359] In Alzheimer's disease, the olfactory system is even more directly involved; virtually all the primarily affected parts of the brain (such as the medial group of amygdaloid nuclei) have connections with the generally seriously degenerated olfactory bulbus.[360] Deterioration in the field of smell therefore might trigger damage to the brain as a whole. Similarly, in patients with dementia in the form of Alzheimer's disease, the capacity for smell, after an initial decline, remains relatively stable, while other functions continue to decline (such as hearing and sight, as measured with a Picture Identification Test, or PIT).[361] Noradrenaline, an important neurotransmitter, likewise shows a greatly reduced concentration in the olfactory bulbus of elderly people with dementia, patients suffering from Korsakoff's psychosis and those suffering from Parkinson's disease, meaning that the synaptic contact between the nerve cells takes place either slowly or not at all.[362]

It is conceivable that Alzheimer's disease is furthered by declining resistance to the chronic "bombardment" of toxic substances in the nasal cavities, which can also find their way through the olfactory epithelium into the nerve fiber of the brain.[363] It is well known that certain substances—sulphuric acid, for example—have a devastating effect on the sense of smell itself. It is possible that, given the replacement process of sensory cells (see Chapter 2), toxic substances are eventually taken further and further toward the brain, with the concomitant results. It recently emerged that people who have had a long period of schooling have a lower chance of developing this kind of dementia. That fact need not have anything to do with the education itself; it is quite conceivable that those with a high level of education were less exposed to harmful odors, if only because they belonged to a higher social class. If this line of thought is correct, Alzheimer's disease is therefore caused in part by a decline in the sense of smell and through the "dragging" of toxic substances in the direction of the brain. The following fact is important in these processes.

According to epidemiological research, smokers are less likely than non-smokers to develop Alzheimer's disease. As we saw previously (Chapter 4), nicotine has a certain protective function for the olfactory organ. If degeneration of the sense of smell does indeed go together with the emergence of this kind of dementia, it is conceivable that smokers are less likely to contract the disease. But whatever the case, a relatively rapidly deteriorating sense of smell may be of important supplementary diagnostic value in determining a general process of dementia.

In Alzheimer's disease two phases are distinguished; the patients' sense of smell in phase II is no worse than in phase I, which means that the decline in the sense of smell takes place early in the pathological process. Subsequently, the sense of smell does not change any more than it does among healthy people of the same age. In short, the beginnings of decay in phylogenetically older parts of the brain—perhaps leading to or contributing to Alzheimer's disease—do not continue in those areas; hence decay remains limited. The emotional disorders also observed are probably caused by the elimination from the neocortex of increasing numbers of cognitive control systems that help to determine the functioning of the limbic system.[364]

The situation is not a simple one, however. Patients suffering from Korsakoff's psychosis—a disease resembling dementia which often occurs in middle age as a result of alcoholism and particularly malnutrition (specifically, it is a deficiency of the vitamin B complex)—have a severely reduced capacity for smell compared with healthy people of the same age. Many old people with dementia, in contrast, still smell reasonably well, provided account is taken of their reduced intelligence in testing.[365] Here the same kind of communication problem presents itself as with investigating toddlers. It is unfruitful to ask an elderly person with dementia for his or her impressions—he or she will have forgotten them in an instant—so facial expressions (frowning, smiling, yawning, turning the nose up) and about twenty other kinds of behavior are used to map the olfactory and taste experience of patients with dementia.[366] It is striking that old people with dementia smell and taste more or less like normal people of the same age. Olfactory and taste stimuli, however, lead to longer-lasting reactions with these people; the decreased capacity for smell therefore has proportionately more effect on behavior.

These considerations and facts also pose the question of how worthwhile the lives of our fellow human beings with dementia are. Perhaps we underestimate the positive aspects of being thrown back into a confined space. Are we healthy people not too fixated on the wide world of eyes and ears, language and intellect, which is full of stimuli? Isn't the demented person with all his handicaps and loneliness—like the naive little child—also able to enjoy what is close, what is small-scale, what is essential? Old people with dementia, for example, have a very pregnant use of language. They question the value of status, intelligence and possessions, and the nuanced expressions of emotions; they regard laughing together and enjoying a cigarette as more important. Perhaps those with dementia are in a certain sense just as original as people who are mentally healthy. "Bystanders constantly try to bring him or her back to reality. Our reality. Then they get irritable: good gracious, can't you remember that? That's logical, but it is not the right approach. You'd do better to try to empathize with their world, to follow them into it as far as possible."[367] Are those with dementia perhaps more fascinated by concrete, close and non-intellectual stimuli because the neocortex as a whole is now playing a much less dominant role? And what is wrong with that?

Aromatherapy

Since there is an oblique connection with the subject of this chapter, we would like to say a few words about the increasing popularity of "aromatherapies," which are used (albeit still on a limited scale) in the treatment of both mental and physical ailments.[368]

Homer advised burning sulphur in houses where there were sick people, and Hippocrates proposed combating the plague with the aid of burning brushwood, a practice used as late as the eighteenth century in Marseilles. At home one was supposed to be able to ward off the plague with scented bags containing various herbs. In Europe aromatherapy became popular particularly from the sixteenth century onward. Montaigne, for example, advocated the use—including the medical use—of stimulating smells; he maintained that those odors brought about changes in him which were fairly specifically linked to the odor concerned. Shakespeare had King Lear ask for civet in order to combat his dark moods. The Leiden physician Hermann Boerhaave was convinced that the sick might recover if one were to put naked young girls in their beds; their body odor, he believed, had a regenerative effect, and he is said to have demonstrated this with a German prince. This idea also occurs in the Bible: King David was given the use of a beautiful virgin, who by lying in his bed lengthened his life. A doctor once announced in a scientific tome that regenerative "apoplectic balsams" spread in the brain, where they were able to thin the mucus and other juices, so that vital spirits located in the brain were stimulated and set in motion.[369] Finally, nervous people were absurdly advised to smell flowers; because flowers have no nervous system, their smells were supposed to have calming effects.

Nowadays advocates of aromatherapy maintain that inhaled odors and oils absorbed through the skin affect one's hormonal balance, physical resistance to disease and the central nervous system—an argument which is not incorrect. According to some researchers, many odors also affect the frequency of one's breathing, blood pressure, electrical resistance of the skin and the contingent negative variation (CNV) of the EEG, the electrical phenomenon that indicates one's degree of alertness or wakefulness.[370] Following are a few examples of the use of smells and essences in this kind of therapy, with the caveat that the research conducted is generally not very impressive.

Musk is said to be effective for melancholy. Basil, peppermint, rose, neroli (an oil distilled from orange blossom) and cloves are supposed to enhance wakefulness. Sandalwood, marjoram (oregano), bergamot oil, camomile and lemon, on the other hand, are supposed to encourage relaxation. Lavender is supposed to have an effect on asthma, eczema, insomnia and anxiety phenomena. Peppermint is said to be an effective remedy for mental exhaustion, pain, nausea and intestinal disorders. The rose is used in cases of depression, hangovers, impotence and frigidity, and the smell of sandalwood is very useful when someone is suffering from inflammation of the throat. Rose essence is supposed to benefit the liver, the stomach and the blood; an antidepressive effect is also ascribed to this substance. Jasmine essence is—because of the pheromone-like substances it contains?—sometimes used as a general tonic, and essence of the white lotus flower is supposed to combat coughing. Other smells have varying effects. The smell of a geranium calms one person, but makes another nervous.

Aromatherapies, some people claim, are used with varying success to combat addiction and depression.[371] One of the uses involves linking the patient's attention to smells during therapy. It is claimed that outside the therapeutic situation the inhaling of those smells evokes an atmosphere or general mood which stops the patient from reaching for the bottle or hypodermic syringe. Attention or "empathy" is an important component of psychotherapy; it is conceivable that a feeling of "being given attention" via conditioning to an odor can be evoked again.

Nothing is more relaxing than taking a bath at 90 degrees Fahrenheit while listening to the breaking surf on headphones, and feasting your eyes on wonderful fantasy figures. With this in mind, a special apparatus has been developed, called a floater: a fiberglass bathtub in which you are enclosed as in a cocoon. Epsom salts are dissolved in the water, allowing you to lie bobbing up and down in a virtually weightless state. People who float in this way appear to lose their sense of time; they say that it reduces stress and acts as a painkiller as well.[372] The smell of the sea (which perhaps recalls amniotic fluid) is also supposed to be relaxing and is therefore also used in aromatherapy.[373]

The New Age movement can perhaps be understood as acting out a longing for the pristine first impressions of the fetal state. Are people looking for birth in the New Age? They appear to be. In that case, the New Age movement should adopt a salmon as a logo, because (as we observed earlier) this fish returns to its breeding grounds after a period at sea—often streams and rivulets far inland where the creature spent its young days. There are indications that the salmon has imprinted the smells of those rivulets, so that they function as a kind of compass.[374]

Chapter 9

Conclusion

The environment we enter at birth is a fog bank, a confused whole or a cloud of atoms, which gradually is transformed into a world with a structure. We have no idea what to do, and we give voice to our helplessness by starting to cry. In order to survive, we constantly have to react in meaningful ways to the environment; from it we excavate the raw materials with which to enhance our personal well-being. This means that we constantly have to judge the environment on its merits. In the "buzzing, blooming confusion"—as the psychologist William James described the world of the young child over a century ago—we have to learn to distinguish between what is important to us and what is unimportant. Senses are essential tools for that purpose; they provide the material necessary for us to discern a structure in the world. The use of the senses has of necessity something forced about it. If a bird is attacked repeatedly by a wasp as it forages for food, all black-and-yellow flies will arouse its suspicions, even though there are edible species among them. For survival, the "nuanced truth" is of little importance; if you are hungry enough, the statutes of the animal rights movement won't seem to matter very much.

The Basic Function of the Sense of Smell

Of all the senses, smell probably best meets the basic function of a sense: making a distinction between *me* and *not me*, as well as between what is relevant and what is irrelevant. It is inevitable that mistakes should be made in such a process, a phenomenon that we find throughout the animal kingdom. Again, ducklings, which come into the world almost as helpless as human beings, follow the first moving object they perceive, on the not unreasonable assumption that it is their mother. If the object is a human being, the duckling regards it as a parent and one of its own species, and once it has grown up the creature even tries to court other human beings.

Doubt is a sign of intelligence: when we hesitate, we put off following a rule without question due to our suspicion that there may be important exceptions. Only through doubt does it emerge that not all flies with black and yellow markings are wasps, and that the creature up ahead is a very strange kind of duck. In nature, however, there is seldom time to collect all the information needed to make decisions. Generally it is necessary to act *quickly*; a rabbit that smells a suspicious smell had better not start a discussion group in order to talk it over: the creature must take flight.

In man, the sense of smell is an important aid in coming to quick decisions. Smell often does not wait for the judgment of the reflective, intellectual powers, but switches immediately to the brain centers that govern behavior. Often these reactions are connected with our emotional interests; they can be described in general terms as "continuing," "stopping," "good" and "bad."[375] The nose doesn't play politics and is made impatient by red tape. The nose tends not to give precedence to the intellect, since delay can be disastrous.

From this it is also possible to understand why there are only a few neutral smells that we perceive consciously in everyday life. That kind of information is generally not important; when we smell something, it is usually something unpleasant or pleasant. In other words, smell is a sense which is decidedly hedonic and linked to emotional life; we often assess in a single sniff whether or not something is important to us. With images and sounds, in contrast, there is a large neutral area, which through experience gains color and meaning in a much more nuanced way; moreover, the eye and the ear focus on a world which is less dominated by the necessity of making a decision quickly.

Although the olfactory organ tends to make mistakes and in certain respects is more subject to illusions than the other senses, it is striking that both man and animals find the messages from the sense of smell reliable and accept them with little doubt: when you smell a smell, you assume something significant is giving it off. A corollary of this function of smell is that the capacity for imagining smells is limited.

People who are concerned with smells on a daily basis (perfumers and those who monitor the smell and taste of products) maintain that they can imagine smells easily, but that is true only in a limited way.[376] Generally our memories of a smell and of the context in which it played a role emerge only when we smell it again. You can imagine your old nursery school—the look and sound of the classroom—but what can you remember of the smells that hung around it? Everyone knows the smell of pine needles, but the detail with which you can imagine a pine tree (and possibly draw it) is matched by the dreariness or emptiness of its smell when you imagine it. We have to bring the tree into the house and smell it properly. The fact that we do this at Christmas might be connected with the fact that the smell of pine needles reduces stress and aggression and anxiety and during holidays particularly tensions between people threaten to erupt.

Although we can to a certain extent learn to smell better or differently, it is difficult to shake off our dislike of a particular smell. Such forms of conditioning take place rapidly and are very persistent. Research has shown that a neutral smell, given off in some situation or other, very quickly becomes a marker for the circumstances. The result of this may be that the smell in another context leads to reactions appropriate to the original circumstances.[377] If you've racked your brains over an impossible puzzle in a room full of a strange smell, you may feel the fear of failure if you smell that smell again somewhere else. The smell of kerosene will have a fatal influence on your peace of mind if you've ever been in a flying accident, even though other sensory signals try to convince you that there is no cause for concern. In brief, once you've made a judgment linked to a smell, that judgment tends to stick. You can get used to a smell, but this happens due to adaptation or habituation: you no longer smell the smell consciously. We get used to the effects of smells on our emotional life and behavior much less quickly; moreover, we may react only at a physical level to an adapted or weak smell. Considering all the unpleasant associations smells can evoke, we might say that anosmic people are lucky.

Apart from the wide interpersonal and intrapersonal differences in the capacity to distinguish and appreciate smells, messages from the olfactory organ are interpreted objectively to the extent that what we smell we must be able to trace in the environment. At least we have a higher expectation of this with smells than with images or sounds. We do not consider the stars we see when we get up in a hurry as a whim of the environment: we blame them on low blood pressure or some such. When we hear ringing in our ears, we don't think mice are singing to us, but that blood vessels in the ear have become constricted or been damaged by a loud noise. The sources of the smells that we smell, on the other hand, are projected outside the olfactory organ; we seldom think of a kind of delusion or a delicate condition of the sense of smell itself or of the body to which the nose belongs.

It is well known, however, that old people quite commonly suffer from olfactory hallucinations. There are various causes for this. Sometimes it is a result of an *arteria vertebralis* that functions less well because of "collapsing" vertebrae in the neck, which supplies part of our brain with blood. Loss of smell plays into the hands of smell hallucinations.[378] And we know that olfactory sensory cells display spontaneous activity: even in a virtually odorless environment they transmit signals to the brain, so it is possible for a person to report a smell which is not there. Suggestion plays an important part in this. It must be noted that this is different from imagining a particular smell; people who participate in an olfactory research project expect to have to smell *something*.

An anecdote in this area.[379] During a lecture a researcher asked the students if they would participate in an experiment to demonstrate the speed of diffusion of a substance in space. To do this properly, a pungent chemical had to be used, he said. The researcher took a bottle out of a box lined with cotton wool, carefully unscrewed the top, dabbed the contents on a cotton cloth and, averting his face, pointed the strip in the direction of the students. As soon as the students smelled something, they were to raise their hands to show that the "wave front" of the smell had been perceived. The students in the front row put up their hands quite quickly, and following that the smell front moved on. Three-quarters of the students perceived the smell, which they found unpleasant, and the others probably would have smelled it too, but the experiment had to be abandoned because several students in the front rows became nauseous and asked to leave the lecture hall. At that point the researcher considered it appropriate to tell them that the "pungent chemical" the cloth had been sprinkled with was water.

• • •

We shall conclude with a number of tips and observations.

General Characteristics

- The impression made by a smell is heavily dependent on the concentration of the substance; stinking substances may even come to smell pleasant in a low concentration.
- People wanting to smell as much as possible should crawl on the ground or lie on the floor during meetings.
- It is conceivable that a smell makes a slightly different impression on us depending on which nostril we inhale it through.
- Unconsciously influenced by a smell, we may be prompted to do or avoid doing or feeling something without fully understanding why.

- Smells can cause fairly radical physical changes without our realizing it.
- We are less likely to have unconscious physical reactions to smells if we are able to name the smells.
- Smells are generally difficult to express in language, because the olfactory organ has connections mainly with sections of the brain that are old in evolutionary terms and not involved directly in language systems and with the right hemisphere of the brain. For similar reasons we generally have trouble imagining smells.
- If you smell a fire, you're better off sniffing briefly a number of times rather than inhaling the air in one long breath. If you are not sure whether what you smell is a fire, go outside for a moment to give the olfactory organ a chance to recover, then go back inside and smell again.
- The short-term olfactory memory has a "recognition peak" at approximately twelve seconds.
- If it is necessary to determine the direction a smell is coming from, inhale *briefly* and turn your head from side to side.
- Odorants appear to have greater intensity if they are colored.
- Sometimes a foul stench can be combated by adding a small quantity of a stinking substance to the mixture. One stench may mask another. Conversely, adding a substance that smells pleasant can make the stench worse; so can adding an odorless substance.
- If you're an employer, beware of buildings with air conditioning and windows that cannot be opened. Such buildings are often filled with a non-locatable and indefinable stench, which chronically irritates people and to some extent alarms them, making them less productive and prone to call in sick.
- It is sensible not to talk much during meals and not to smoke. Talking with one's mouth full is not only bad manners; it also makes you taste less, because the smells of the food penetrate the olfactory organ through the oral cavity. Smoking, of course, reduces the sensitivity of the olfactory organ.
- When eating, do not mix the different foods together, but

take successive mouthfuls of each, in order to prevent habituation and loss of sensitivity of one's smell and taste.

- Do not sniff at the food too much before eating; just smelling can lead to a completely different perception than allowing smell and taste to work in parallel by eating.

Individual Differences

- Generally speaking, thirty-year-olds have the best olfactory memory.
- Smell specialists, such as perfumers, smell scarcely better than other people, although they often claim to smell uncommonly well.
- Blind people do not smell better than sighted people.
- Compared with other senses, there are enormous differences in the olfactory capacity among people.
- Smokers smell relatively poorly; if you give up smoking, it may take several months for you to recover the capacity to smell.
- Inhaling cocaine, glue or sulphuric acid can seriously damage the sense of smell.
- Elderly people are advised to add some artificial taste and smell additives to their food. (Those who manage old people's homes, nursing institutions, hospitals and the like, take note.)
- Old people often suffer from olfactory hallucinations.

Men and Women

- Generally speaking, women smell better than men.
- If you can't tell whether food has spoiled, have a woman decide rather than a man.
- If a name has to be given to a smell, ask a woman rather than a man.
- During menstruation, women smell relatively poorly.
- Male sweat extract can have some influence on the regularity of a woman's menstrual cycle.

- On average, men have a more pungent body odor than women, and their breath is more unpleasant.
- If you grow a mustache, you'll smell both pleasant and unpleasant smells longer than usual.

Mood and Performance

- Smell is a special sense to the extent that odors influence the brain, the hormonal system, and behavior generally. Conversely, the brain and many physical processes influence smell.
- As much as possible, breathe through your nose and not through your mouth. For many reasons, breathing through the nose is better for the functioning of the body as a whole. Besides, you'll smell better through the nose and this will improve your mood, concentration and general well-being (in children, too).
- There is a rhythm of approximately three hours in the penetrability of the nostrils. When the right nostril is open, there is a relatively great amount of activity in the left hemisphere (language, thought); an open left nostril corresponds with a relatively great amount of activity in the right hemisphere (including spatial representation and the experience of emotions).
- Smells basically evoke two reactions: an intellectual reaction and an emotional reaction (behavior, that is). Since the right hemisphere is strongly activated in smelling, the emotional reaction to an odor may dominate.
- Alertness can be both heightened and lowered by smells.
- Smells can influence mood.
- Smells sometimes have some effect on one's performance at work, one's inclinations in the marketplace and one's tendencies toward aggression and anxiety.
- The smell in a bedroom (a child's bedroom, too) can either improve or disrupt the quality of one's sleep.
- Smells characteristically evoke memories (emotional or otherwise) of events long since forgotten.

- If you make your house smell pleasant, not only will you probably feel better but you will remember more pleasant events.
- Feelings of anxiety toward certain circumstances can be linked to a smell that happened to be present at the time they occurred. Avoid that smell, because smelling it in other situations may evoke irrational fears.
- Many smells are linked with certain colors.

Body Odors

- There are indications that babies in the womb experience smell-like sensations and that these may be important for their later development.
- In general, infants drink better when breast-fed than when bottle-fed, because when breast-feeding they can smell their mother better.
- Children often cry less when their mother's clothing is laid unwashed next to their heads.
- Mothers and children can recognize each other very well on the basis of smell. The same applies to other family members, notably brothers and sisters.
- People can distinguish their own body odor quite well from that of other people.
- One's body odor is to some extent hereditary.
- An instinctive dislike of someone may be connected to their body odor.
- There are considerable cultural and racial differences in the strength of body odor.

Perfumes

- A good perfume gives off three different smells in succession.
- Do not buy cheap perfumes. They are often mixtures whose components have different rates of habituation. The result

may be that the perfume smells pleasant at first but then begins to stink shortly afterward.

- A perfume does not smell the same on everyone, because it interacts chemically with a person's body odor.
- Men often become confused and react negatively toward a woman if she is both perfumed and formally dressed. To a lesser extent women respond that way as well.
- If you have young children, either do not use too much perfume or wear lots of perfume *all the time*. If you use perfume only on special occasions, your children may develop a dislike of it because they associate it with abandonment.

Sex

- It has been claimed that some plants smell like sperm or the female genitalia.
- During puberty, a radical change occurs in the appreciation of all kinds of smells. Girls' sensitivity to smell particularly increases sharply in that period.
- Sexual stimulation can lead to swelling of the nasal mucous membrane and to sneezing.
- There is little evidence that specific sex pheromones are active in man. Pheromone-like substances can, however, have an unconscious influence on bodily and emotional functioning.
- Animal pheromones (whether or not they are incorporated in perfumes) have some influence on the way in which we judge other people.
- To the extent that pheromones affect our actions, those effects are slightly different in men than in women.
- Male pheromone-like substances may have a certain influence on women's moods. These substances are found particularly in armpit sweat and saliva. These substances occur in large concentrations in blacks and to a lesser extent in Asians. It is well known that these so-called androstenes put women in a somewhat "mellow" mood, while repelling men.

- If one shaves one's armpits, pheromones have much less effect.
- Generally speaking, women like aftershave more than men. So whether a man should use aftershave depends on the extent to which he has contact with both sexes.

Olfactory Disorders and Diseases

- The sense of smell often contributes to a depressive state (such as a memory dysfunction), except in the case of innate smell blindness.
- Be careful when painting indoors. Your sense of smell can be permanently damaged, unless you smoke in the intervals between painting.
- If you have an olfactory disorder, do not go to a doctor but to an olfactory specialist. Olfactory problems often resolve themselves spontaneously (though sometimes slowly), but a number of disorders are treatable.
- Olfactory disorders are always connected with taste problems.
- An olfactory disorder *may* indicate a mental or physical disease entirely unconnected with the sense of smell itself.
- Some diseases (including tumors of the hypophysis) result in a considerable increase in one's sensitivity to smell.
- Dementia quite often begins with a decline in the capacity to smell.
- You may have less chance of contracting Alzheimer's disease if you have smoked, since nicotine has a certain protective influence on the olfactory organ.
- Breath odor may give some indication whether a person has a particular disease.
- If someone is no longer able to make a connection between smells that belong together (such as the smell of tobacco and the smell of a burning cigarette), the person may be suffering from damage to the right hemisphere of the brain.
- Certain drugs influence the functioning of the sense of smell

in a negative way. This is true of certain antidepressants, which may make the depressive state worse.

- It is not yet clear whether aromatherapy is truly effective.
- Because smells evoke many emotional associations and memories, hospitals might do well to introduce various smells artificially into the atmosphere.

Notes

1. Good venous pressure in the chest cavity is important for blood circulation as a whole. In addition, inflammation of the middle ear and the sinuses appears to occur less frequently, one's stance becomes more upright, children's ability to concentrate is said to be increased, and so on.
2. Unless otherwise indicated, a large part of this section is taken from the cultural-historical survey by Corbin (1986).
3. Stoddart (1990).
4. The "hearing" of the music of the spheres was called *acroasis*.
5. The idea was not unusual. For example, it was also believed that there was a separate "warmth substance" (*phlogiston*).
6. Stoddart (1990). This kind of idea may already have existed in antiquity. Both Hippocrates and the Roman authors Horace and Juvenal thought that the atmosphere in late summer and autumn often caused fever.
7. This notion is not completely nonsensical, to the extent that harmful substances breathed in through the nose can cause brain damage.
8. This probably also dates back to antiquity. The hospital of Hippocrates and the surgeries of doctors were described as follows. "The atmosphere in the *iatreion* is characterized by a special hospital air: smoke from a stove in which the cauterizing instruments are kept red-hot, the vapors of boiling medicines, the aroma of herbs, resins and spices on the shelves and a touch of roasted human flesh." In Hoes (1994).
9. Roman bathing had three stages. In the *unctuarium* one perfumed oneself with scents, the *frigidarium* was for cooling off, and finally one entered

the *tepidarium*, the warm bath, where one was scrubbed down by a slave.

10. See Vroon & Draaisma (1986). At about the same time the first book on an "unconscious mental life" by C. G. Carus appeared.

11. Stoddart (1990).

12. Quotes taken from Corbin (1986).

13. See, e.g., Amoore (1970). In antiquity this idea was advanced by Lucretius.

14. Köster (1971).

15. In Corbin (1986).

16. A. P. J. Hendriks, unpublished research.

17. Stoddart (1990).

18. See, e.g., Engen (1982).

19. Wallraff (1990).

20. Sheldrake (1994). It is still not known by what mechanism homing pigeons are able to find their way back to their loft. Recent experiments were carried out at the University of Utrecht with a loft whose location had been changed. The pigeons were found to alight where the loft had *previously* stood. And if earlier that loft had been in other places, these were visited first before the pigeons looked further. So the smell of the loft probably plays no major part in the pigeons' homing behavior.

21. "Limbic" comes from *limbus*, strip or band. The reference is to a number of structures which are, as it were, wrapped around the brain stem.

22. An exception is so-called limbic language, or cries of fear, disgust and pain. These cries probably derive from the limbic system (see Vroon, 1992). As far as emotions are concerned, there is a "fast" and a "slow" processing route in the central nervous system. The fast route results in a stimulus leading immediately to an emotional response, so that in retrospect the person is often surprised at his or her own behavior.

23. Corbin (1986), Jerison (1982).

24. For a discussion of this point, see Roede et al. (1991); the aquatic-man hypothesis is vigorously defended by Morgan (1990).

25. Hepper (1987).

26. Gibbons (1986), Stoddart (1990).

27. Costanzo & Graziadei (1987).

28. The principal sources used for this section are: Costanzo & Graziadei (1987), Engen (1982), Lancet (1986), Macrides et al. (1985), Moran et al. (1991), Mozell (1971), Price (1985, 1987), Scott & Harrison (1987), Shipley & Reyes (1991), Stoddart (1990).

29. See Van Toller et al. (1985).

30. You can duplicate this as follows. Draw a star on a piece of paper and put an arbitrary number of dots around it. Stare at the star: after a while a number of dots will suddenly disappear (the Troxler effect).

31. Mozell et al. (1969), discussed in Engen (1982).

32. From: Engen (1982).

33. This phenomenon is called intermodal interaction; it applies to all the senses to a certain extent.
34. Snyder et al. (1989).
35. Moran et al. (1991).
36. In this book various animal experiments are described which according to current opinion are ethically reprehensible. However, in view of the fact that they have been carried out, there is little point in ignoring the results.
37. Stoddart (1990).
38. Claassen (1993).
39. Lancet (1986).
40. Doty et al. (1981); see also Chapter 6.
41. From Carr et al. (1990).
42. See, e.g., Shipley (1985).
43. Anholt (1987).
44. Farbman (1990).
45. Moran et al. (1991).
46. Debagge et al. (1982), Gibbons (1986), Gonzales & Farbman (1984).
47. Morrison & Graziadei (1983), Costanzo & Graziadei (1987).
48. The following two sections are quite technical in content; the reader may wish to skip them or go through them quickly. Some of the sources consulted are: Carr et al. (1990), Chastrette & Zakarya (1991), Getchell & Getchell (1987, 1991), Korsching (1991), Lancet (1986), Lancet & Pace (1987), Margolis (1985), Pace et al. (1985), Price (1984), Sicard & Holley (1984), Snyder et al. (1988, 1989).
49. Lancet established nine criteria on this point (1986); there is no scope here to list them.
50. Price (1984).
51. Gibbons (1986), Tisserand (1988). The principle applies to other senses, to the extent that covering the eyes and ears of newborn children leads to deafness and blindness.
52. From: Freeman (1991), see also Macrides et al. (1985), Scott & Harrison (1987).
53. Shipley & Reyes (1991).
54. Sicard & Holley (1984), Kauer (1987).
55. See Kauer (1987) for a theoretical model.
56. Haberly & Bower (1989), Freeman (1991).
57. Price (1985, 1987).
58. Shipley & Reyes (1991).
59. Keverne et al. (1986), Silver (1987).
60. Wysocki & Meredith (1987).
61. Cain & Murphy (1980).
62. Silver (1987).
63. Wysocki & Meredith (1987).

64. Stoddart (1990).
65. Stuiver (1958).
66. Some names and publications that can be mentioned in this connection are Koelega (1980) and Köster (1971) at the University of Utrecht (where the olfactory research department was closed down in the 1980s). At the Agricultural University of Wageningen (e.g., Schiet & Frijters, 1988) and the Unilever Research Laboratory in Vlaardingen (Overbosch, 1986), research is being carried out in the field of the psychophysics of smell and taste.
67. Corbin (1986).
68. See Engen (1982), Stoddart (1990). *Hēdonē* is Greek for pleasure or enjoyment.
69. See *The Flora of Heukels & Van Ooststroom* (1977).
70. *La fleur de châtaignier*, paraphrased in Stoddart (1990).
71. Doty (1991a).
72. Henning (1924).
73. See, e.g., Köster (1971).
74. Arctander (1969), Chastrette et al. (1988).
75. Amoore (1970). This notion was put forward in antiquity by Lucretius. It also exists in the field of pharmacology: it is thought that drugs attach on the basis of their shape to "holes" in cell membranes.
76. See also Geldard (1972).
77. Chastrette & Zakarya (1991), Ohloff (1986).
78. Pike et al. (1988).
79. Vroon, unpublished research.
80. Marks et al. (1988).
81. The "signal detection theory" is used for this; see Doty (1991a).
82. Warren et al. (1992).
83. Rabin & Cain (1986).
84. Engen (1982).
85. Stevens et al. (1988).
86. Cometto-Muñiz & Cain (1990).
87. See Köster (1971) and Köster & De Wijk (1991).
88. See, e.g., Cain & Polak (1992), Köster (1971).
89. Engen (1982).
90. Cain (1977); see also Köster & De Wijk (1991).
91. Slotnick & Pazos (1990).
92. Cain (1977). Köster (1971) mentions no fewer than seven possible localizations of the adaptation process which he is unable to decide among.
93. Borroni & Atema (1988).
94. Gross-Isseroff & Lancet (1988).
95. See Corbin (1986). It is said that aphrodisiacs do not exist. That is not completely true. The adrenal gland makes, for example, the substance dehydroxy-epi-androsterone (usually referred to as DHEA), a predecessor of male and female sex hormones. High consumption of that substance in-

creases the sexual urge (and protects one against cardiovascular diseases and cancer).

96. Of course, there is an alarm for sulphuric acid in the control room, but it is tuned to such a degree of sensitivity that the staff switch it off.
97. Van Toller et al. (1985), Mennella & Beauchamp (1991).
98. See Engen (1982), Enns & Hornung (1985), Laing (1991).
99. Murphy (1987).
100. Köster, in: Wagenaar, Vroon & Janssen (1978).
101. Mozell (1971).
102. Laing & Willcox (1983).
103. Laing & Francis (1989).
104. Laing & MacLeod (1992).
105. Laing & Glemarec (1992).
106. Laska & Hudson (1992).
107. Laing & Willcox (1983).
108. Morgan (1990).
109. The aquatic-man hypothesis does not accord very well with the fact that changing passability of the nostrils also occurs in rats that do not enter the water. (Stoddart, 1990).
110. See Vroon (1992) for a list of examples. According to Stephen Jay Gould: "Remnants of the past that don't make sense in present terms—the useless, the odd, the peculiar, the incongruous—are the signs of history." This phenomenon is even more mysterious if one realizes that in smelling it is mainly the right hemisphere which is active. The observation mentioned was made while the test subjects were not smelling anything in particular. It would be interesting to investigate what happens when odors are smelled continuously: depending on the nostril, these smells may have a somewhat different quality.
111. The alternating and forced breathing through one nostril has long been known to the theory of yoga.
112. Kobal et al. (1989).
113. Laing & MacLeod (1992), Freeman (1991).
114. In the case of sight the phenomenon is called lateral inhibition, with the difference that it occurs within one retina.
115. Doty (1991b).
116. Hepper (1987).
117. Teicher & Blass (1977).
118. Mennella & Beauchamp (1991).
119. Doty (1991b).
120. Lipsitt et al., in: Schaal (1988).
121. Engen (1982).
122. Schmidt & Beauchamp (1988).
123. Mennella & Beauchamp (1991).
124. Schaal (1988).

125. O'Connell et al. (1989).
126. See his book *Cato maior de senectute*.
127. Doty et al. (1984), Eskenazi et al. (1986).
128. Stevens & Cain (1985), Stevens et al. (1989, 1990).
129. For the effect of these ailments on the functioning of breathing and smell, see DeLong & Getchell (1987).
130. Doty (1991c).
131. Enns & Hornung (1988), see also Doty (1991c), Smith & Seiden (1991).
132. Stevens & Cain (1986).
133. Schiffmann (1977).
134. A well-known flavor enhancer is monosodium glutamate. However, many people cannot tolerate this substance and react to it with flushing, agitation, palpitations and insomnia.
135. Doty (1991a). However, this fact is somewhat controversial. If one compares smokers and non-smokers using only one or a few substances, the difference is not very great. However, this may be due to the fact that repeated acquaintance with the same smell lowers the threshold value— that is, a kind of learning effect.
136. Mair & Harrison (1991).
137. Doty (1991a).
138. Schwartz (1991). The research concentrated mainly on the influence of the quality of the air on the capacity to smell of various employees in a paint factory. The concentrations given in the table are comparable with the air that painters breathe in when working outside, in a large building, and indoors, respectively.
139. Edwards et al. (1987).
140. Doty (1991a).
141. Doty et al. (1982), Doty (1990). We shall return to this point.
142. Doty et al. (1985).
143. For this test, see also Chapter 8.
144. Cain (1982).
145. The French olfactory researcher J. Le Magnen once toyed with the idea of using the varying sensitivity to smell of the woman as an aid in the rhythm method of birth control. However, this method is very unreliable and can, for example, be interfered with by a cold.
146. In some cultures there are only three words or so to designate colors. In the laboratory, however, it appears that these people can distinguish many more shades. Apart from that, it has been shown the differences between left and right are strongly linked to the acquired direction of reading and writing; see Zwaan (1965).
147. Doty (1991b), Davis & Pangborn (1985).
148. Schleidt et al. (1988).
149. See Freeland (1980), who has demonstrated this for the mangabey.
150. Schleidt et al. (1988).

151. See Schab (1991).
152. Stoddart (1990).
153. Lorig et al. (1988).
154. Van Toller, in: Tisserand (1988).
155. Badia et al. (1990).
156. Lorig & Schwartz (1988).
157. Freeman & Grajski (1987).
158. Freeman (1991).
159. It has, however, been noted that there are nerves which run from the brain *to* the retina and that the retina contains receptors for benzodiazepines (sedatives). However, as yet we have no understanding of the associated processes.
160. Kucharski & Hall (1987).
161. There are various cross-connections between the hemispheres. The largest one is the *corpus callosum*; two smaller ones are the *commissura anterior* and the *commissura posterior*.
162. The brain stem, for example, has had more or less the same functions for hundreds of millions of years and is scarcely capable of learning. See also Vroon (1992).
163. Tisserand (1988).
164. For a historical survey of this discussion, see Harrington (1987) and Blakeslee (1980).
165. Abraham & Mathai (1983).
166. Van Toller, in: Tisserand (1988).
167. Staubli et al. (1987).
168. Hvastja & Zanuttini (1989).
169. Richardson & Zucco (1989).
170. Schab (1991).
171. Frijda (1988).
172. Murphy & Cain (1986).
173. Rabin (1988).
174. Van Toller et al. (1983).
175. Rabin & Cain (1984), Lyman & McDaniel (1986).
176. Schab (1991).
177. Jelicic (1992).
178. Walk & Johns (1984), Lyman & McDaniel (1986, 1990).
179. Engen (1982), Richard & Zucco (1989).
180. See also Vroon (1987, 1992). It is sometimes claimed that the linguistic system of the right hemisphere is comparable to that of a two- or three-year-old child.
181. Engen (1987).
182. Schab & Cain (1991).
183. Schab (1990); however, see also Lyman & McDaniel (1990), who did find an effect.

184. Schab & Cain (1991).
185. Barker & Weaver (1983).
186. Walk & Johns (1984).
187. Schab & Cain (1991).
188. Rabin & Cain (1984).
189. Baddeley (1990).
190. Raaijmakers (1993).
191. In the case of sexual abuse, it may even happen that a huge series of (satanic) scenes is imagined. See La Fontaine (1994).
192. Herz & Cupchik (1992); see also Rubin et al. (1984).
193. Ehrlichman & Halpern (1988).
194. Smith et al. (1992).
195. Cann & Ross (1989).
196. Kirk-Smith et al. (1983).
197. That women perform slightly worse in these kinds of tasks is connected with another general fact: on average women have a slightly better and faster language development; generally speaking, the man has a slightly better-developed spatial sense.
198. Tisserand (1988).
199. Ludvigson & Rottman (1989).
200. Claassen (1993).
201. Based on reports in the *Volkskrant* of 22 March 1993, p. 2, and of 14 November 1992 (supplement, "100 years of psychology"); see also *Intermediair* of 29 January 1993, p. 39.
202. In: Corbin (1986). However, we must bear in mind, in regard to the activating influence which smells have on episodic memory, that the effect of visual and auditory stimuli has been less researched or been given less attention. What would happen to someone's memory capacity if they were allowed to hear the sounds of their nursery school fifty years later? Van den Berg and Van Reekum conducted a study which is (obliquely) connected with this (1994). If one combines a hedonically neutral stimulus with a stimulus which is regarded as strongly positive or negative, the appreciation shifts from the neutral stimulus to the positive or to the negative side (conditioning). The researchers linked neutral pictures to unknown smells and then unfamiliar sounds. On the basis of the notion that smells also have mainly hedonic qualities, it was anticipated that the smells would have more influence on the pictures than on the sounds. Actually, smells produced a more *positive* conditioning effect on the appreciation of the pictures, independent of the question whether the smells were found to be neutral, pleasant or unpleasant.
203. Engen (1982).
204. Zellner & Kautz (1990).
205. That diffuse network also exists in the motor system. The newborn infant

has billions of direct links between the cortex and the spinal cord, which are subsequently almost all severed.

206. This has been established by means of a PET scan (positron-emission tomography).
207. Corbin (1986) describes a period in which the language is, as it were, deodorized.
208. See Rindisbacher (1993) for a selection, and Corbin (1986).
209. Fragment taken from Corbin (1986).
210. *Mulier tum bene olet, ubi nihil olet.*
211. *Postume, non bene olet, qui bene semper olet.* Less loosely translated: "After death a person who was always well perfumed no longer smells sweet."
212. Freeman (1991), Tisserand (1988).
213. This phenomenon also means that we often make decisions in an extremely strange way. See, e.g., Nisbett & Ross (1980).
214. Van Toller, research described in Tisserand (1988).
215. Vroon (1990a).
216. Toxins linked to certain microorganisms may play a part in this syndrome. On the other hand, such substances are also present in abundance in domestic kitchens, without producing complaints.
217. Television program *Van gewest tot gewest*, 15 December 1992.
218. Radio program *Aardse zaken*, 5 January 1993.
219. Epple (1974), McClintock (1983), Izard (1983).
220. McClintock (1971).
221. Russell (1983), Preti et al. (1986).
222. First observed in mice in 1955, described in McClintock (1983). In antiquity, moreover, it was thought that sexual abstinence caused women to smell (Corbin, 1986).
223. Cabanac (1971).
224. Engen (1988).
225. Doty (1991a, 1991b, 1991c).
226. Tisserand (1988).
227. Hinde (1983), Te Boekhorst (1991).
228. Stoddart (1990).
229. Simerly (1990), Stoddart (1990).
230. Stoddart (1990).
231. Wilson & Bossert (1963).
232. Calvin (1990).
233. Karlson & Lüscher (1959), Gower et al. (1988), Stoddart (1990). Sex pheromones also play a significant part in amphibians (toads) and reptiles (salamanders); we, however, are restricting the discussion.
234. Isolated by Jacobson et al. (1960).
235. Schneider (1969).
236. Von Frisch (1950).

237. Observation by A.v.A.
238. Stamp Dawkins (1993) even wonders quite seriously whether many birds and mammals have a consciousness.
239. See, e.g., Beauchamp et al. (1976), in: Vandenbergh (1983).
240. Stoddart (1990).
241. See, e.g., Brooksbank et al. (1974), Michael et al. (1971, 1974).
242. Comfort (1971).
243. Stoddart (1990).
244. *Ne trux caper iret in alas.*
245. This phenomenon was first described by K. M. Schneider in 1930. See Stahlbaum & Houpt (1989). Moreover, Virgil wrote in antiquity: "Do you not see how a trembling passes through the body of the horses when they sniff even a whiff of a familiar smell?" (in: Stoddart, 1990).
246. Izard (1983).
247. Meredith (1983).
248. Keverne et al. (1986).
249. Bronson & Macmillan (1983).
250. Michael et al. (1966), Michael & Keverne (1968).
251. Curtis et al. (1971).
252. Corbin (1986).
253. Michael et al. (1974).
254. Filsinger & Fabes (1985).
255. Köster (1986); however, this experiment was not published.
256. Gibbons (1986).
257. There are several thousand rhythms in human behavior which we have not discussed here. Seeing in color, to mention just one example, is best at full moon and in January.
258. Gower et al. (1988).
259. Claus & Alsing (1976), Gower (1984), Gower et al. (1985).
260. Amoore et al. (1977), Wysocki & Beauchamp (1984).
261. Van Toller (1988).
262. Koelega (1980).
263. Melrose et al. (1974).
264. Claus et al. (1981).
265. Cowley et al. (1977).
266. A suggestion by Filsinger & Fabes (1985).
267. Kirk-Smith et al. (1978).
268. McCollough et al. (1981).
269. Kirk-Smith & Booth (1980).
270. Clark (1978), discussed in Gower et al. (1988).
271. Gustavson et al. (1987).
272. Benton (1982).
273. That, however, is a general fact.

274. McClintock (1983).
275. Whitten et al. (1968).
276. Veith et al. (1983), Cutler et al. (1985).
277. Cutler et al. (1986).
278. Dawkins (1982), Hamilton (1964).
279. See, for example, Gould & Lewontin (1979), Williams (1976).
280. Burley (1979).
281. Turke (1984).
282. Stoddart (1988, 1990).
283. Johnston (1983).
284. In fact, the word "perfume" comes from the Latin *per fumum*, "through smoke" or "what dissolves in smoke."
285. Stoddart (1990). He also mentions an anecdote: a human couple who rubbed musk on their genitals were supposed not to have been able to separate themselves without the help of a considerable quantity of water. One sees a similar phenomenon in dogs, who, unlike human beings, have a bony organ in their penis.
286. Corbin (1986).
287. Corbin (1986). The discovery of photosynthesis in plants also played a part in this.
288. Claassen (1993).
289. See Vroon (1992). Kneissler (1989) looks at this more closely. He mentions a recent "numbing" which is supposed to have happened in our brain because of the many stimuli that we perceive and which we cannot do anything with in our behavior.
290. Van Toller (1988).
291. Le Magnen (1952).
292. Stoddart (1990).
293. Claassen (1993), Stoddart (1990).
294. Stoddart (1990).
295. Van Toller et al. (1985).
296. Le Gros Clark (1952).
297. An example. The English word "self-consciousness" has existed only since the eighteenth century, but no one would dream of denying English people who lived in the sixteenth century self-consciousness. See also Vroon (1992).
298. A distinction is made between analytical, creative and socio-emotional intelligence. These abilities are thought to develop to a considerable extent interdependently, with the blueprint of the socio-emotional intelligence emerging early in life.
299. King (1988).
300. Jessee (1982).
301. See, e.g., Lorenz (1965), Tinbergen (1968).

302. Baron (1981, 1983).
303. A basis for this might be that the two hemispheres of the woman collaborate slightly better than those of the man (Chapter 6).
304. Baron (1986).
305. Based on a report in the "Dag in dag uit" column in the *Volkskrant* of 27 January 1993.
306. Gibbons (1986).
307. Stoddart (1990).
308. Hepper (1988).
309. Lord & Kasprzak (1989).
310. Hold & Schleidt (1977).
311. Doty et al. (1981).
312. Porter et al. (1983).
313. Schaal et al. (1980).
314. Bending of the head and stretching of the arm in small children are linked to each other; this is called the tonic neck reflex.
315. Quoted in Schaal (1988).
316. Porter et al. (1985).
317. Porter et al. (1986).
318. Russell et al. (1983).
319. Alberts (1976), Filsinger & Fabes (1985).
320. Snyder (1977).
321. Schaal (1988).
322. Balogh & Porter (1986).
323. Schaal et al. (1980); see also Cernoch & Porter (1985).
324. MacLean (1990).
325. Doty et al. (1982).
326. For a summary see Doty (1981).
327. Inoculation is rather controversial. There are a number of indications that not having had certain diseases in childhood increases the chance of serious disease later.
328. Katan (1993).
329. It cannot be concluded from the fact that cancer is often *discovered* earlier that the *chances of recovery* have improved since then.
330. See, e.g., Engstrom et al. (1992). However, there has been a recent debate about vitamin C. It is supposed to have been shown by animal experiments that the substance is harmless, and indeed beneficial in a certain dosage. The "turning point" in man is not known (communication from L. Kunst). However, medicine has considerably benefited the *quality* of life.
331. This happened, for example, to the American professor of biology and cancer researcher P. Duesberg and to the discoverer of the virus, L. Montagnier. See Vroon (1993).
332. Smith & Seiden (1991).

333. In: Sacks (1985).
334. Mason et al. (1984).
335. Engen (1982), Van Toller (1988).
336. Even stranger than *blind sight* is Anton's syndrome, in which a person simply denies his or her blindness.
337. Engen (1982), Stoddart (1990).
338. Another possibility is administering the "natural" substance de-hydroxy-epi-androsterone, which was mentioned in Chapter 3; in the body, sex hormones are made from it.
339. Stoddart (1990).
340. Stoddart (1990).
341. Schwartz (1991).
342. Doty et al. (1984).
343. Schwartz (1991).
344. Hendriks (1988), University of Utrecht.
345. As in the degeneration of muscle which occurs when one breaks a leg. When someone is unable, for whatever reason, to walk, "motor programs" in the brain are also affected, with the result that the process of rehabilitation takes a long time.
346. This nerve can for various reasons cease to function in the whole part of the face. In the most serious case this involves a tumor of the so-called bridge corner in the brain.
347. Fahy et al. (1989). The number of theories on anorexia nervosa and bulimia nervosa is, however, very large. See, e.g., Jansen (1990), Tuiten (1993).
348. See Estrum & Renner (1987), reported in: Smith & Seiden (1991).
349. When there is a serious shortage of certain substances there is even "specific hunger," a phenomenon which animals suffer from even more markedly than human beings.
350. See Eslinger et al. (1982), Harrison & Pearson (1989), Smith & Seiden (1991), Schwartz (1991).
351. Of course, this is not the only factor involved in depression. According to Kay (1994), after a "geomagnetic storm" depressive phenomena increase by no less than 36 percent across the whole population. The epiphysis, or pineal gland, seems to be very sensitive to magnetic fields; through this gland the fields might influence the production of neurotransmitters.
352. Doty (1981).
353. A summary of research into the factors which determine personal smell can be found in Schaal (1988), see also Claassen (1993) and Gibbons (1986).
354. *Oral communication* by L. Kunst.
355. Hendriks (1988).
356. Corbin (1986).
357. Engen (1982).
358. It is often claimed that cooking in aluminum pans is a cause of this disease. This is wrong: the aluminum found in "platelets" in the brain is caused by

the normal coloring process in analyzing brain tissue (communication from J. Jolles).

359. Doty (1990).
360. Pearson et al. (1985).
361. Doty et al. (1987).
362. Mair & Harrison (1991).
363. Shipley (1985).
364. This can happen in dramatic form when the *arteria cerebri anterior* is ligated in error in a brain operation. The result is loss of emotional inhibition. See Vroon (1992).
365. Mair et al. (1986).
366. Perl et al. (1992).
367. The *Volkskrant* of 13 November 1993. The interviews quoted here have been collected in: Ingrid H. van Delft (1993), *We komen niet meer waar we geweest zijn. Demente bejaarden aan het woord.* Baarn, Anthos.
368. Stoddart (1990).
369. Corbin (1986).
370. See, e.g., Lawless (1991), Tisserand (1988).
371. King (1988).
372. Based on a report in the *Volkskrant* of 7 April 1993.
373. King (1988).
374. Costanzo & Graziadei (1987).
375. Ornstein & Ehrlich (1989).
376. Experiments with reaction times to words indicate that there is *something* that points to this capacity.
377. Kirk-Smith et al. (1983).
378. Something similar applies to the ability to see. When the retinas are damaged people have the tendency to perceive objects which are not "there." That phenomenon is called palinopsia. Apart from this, it is known that sensory deprivation leads to hallucinations.
379. Engen (1982).

Bibliography

Abraham, A., and K. V. Mathai. "The Effect of Right Temporal Lobe Lesions on Matching of Smells." *Neuropsychologia* 21 (1983): 277–281.

Alberts, J. R. "Olfactory Contributions to Behavioral Development in Rodents." In *Mammalian Olfaction: Reproductive Processes and Behavior*, edited by R. L. Doty. New York: Academic Press, 1976.

Amoore, J. E. *Molecular Basis of Odor*. Springfield, Ill.: Thomas, 1970.

Amoore, J. E., P. Pelosi, and M. J. Forrester. "Specific Anosmias to 5-α-androst-16-en-3-one and ω-pentadecalactone: The Urinous and Musky Primary Odors." *Chemical Senses and Flavour* 2 (1977): 401–425.

Anholt, R. R. H. "Primary Events in Olfactory Reception." *Trends in Biochemical Sciences* 12 (1987): 58–62.

Arctander, S. *Perfume and Flavor Chemicals*. Montclair, N.J., 1969.

Baddeley, A. *Human Memory*. London: Erlbaum, 1990.

Badia, P., N. Wesensten, W. Lammers, J. Culpepper, and J. Harsh. "Responsiveness to Olfactory Stimuli Presented in Sleep." *Physiology and Behavior* 48 (1990): 87–90.

Balogh, R. D., and R. H. Porter. "Olfactory Preferences Resulting from Mere Exposure in Human Neonates." *Infant Behavior and Development* 9 (1986): 395–401.

Barker, L. M., and C. A. Weaver III. "Rapid, Permanent Loss of Memory for Absolute Intensity of Taste and Smell." *Bulletin of the Psychonomic Society* 21 (1983): 281–284.

Baron, R. A. "Olfaction and Human Social Behavior: Effects of a Pleasant Scent on Attraction and Social Perception." *Personality and Social Psychology Bulletin* 7 (1981): 611–616.

——— . "Perfume as a Tactic of Impression Management in Social and Organizational Settings." In *Perfumery: The Psychology and Biology of Fragrance*, edited by S. van Toller and G. H. Dodd. New York: Chapman and Hall, 1988.

——— . "Self-presentation in Job Interviews: When There Can Be 'Too Much of a Good Thing.' " *Journal of Applied Social Psychology* 16 (1986): 16–28.

——— . " 'Sweet Smell of Success?' The Impact of Pleasant Scents on Evaluations of Job Applicants." *Journal of Applied Psychology* 19 (1983): 709–713.

Beauchamp, G. K., R. L. Doty, D. G. Moulton, and R. A. Mugford. "The Pheromone Concept in Mammalian Communication: A Critique." In *Mammalian Olfaction: Reproductive Processes and Behavior*, edited by R. L. Doty. New York: Academic Press, 1976.

Benton, D. "The Influence of Androstenol—a Putative Human Pheromone—on Mood Throughout the Menstrual Cycle." *Biological Psychology* 15 (1982): 249–256.

Berg, H. van den, and C. van Reekum. "Odors, Sounds, and Evaluative Conditioning." Ph.D. diss., Universiteit van Amsterdam, 1994.

Blakeslee, T. R. *The Right Brain*. London: Macmillan, 1980.

Boekhorst, I. J. A. Te. "Social Structure of Three Great Ape Species: An Approach Based on Field Data and Individual Oriented Models." Ph.D. diss., Rijksuniversiteit Utrecht.

Bordewijk, F. *Verzameld werk*. The Hague: Nijgh and Van Ditmar, 1982.

Borroni, P. F., and J. Atema. "Adaptation in Chemoreceptor Cells." *Journal of Comparative Physiology A* 164 (1988): 67–74.

Bronson, F. H., and B. Macmillan. "Hormonal Responses to Primer Pheromones." In *Pheromones and Reproduction in Mammals*, edited by J. G. Vandenbergh. New York: Academic Press, 1983.

Brooksbank, B. W. L., R. Brown, and J. A. Gustafsson. "The Detection of 5-α-androst-16-en-3-α-ol in Human Male Axillary Sweat." *Experientia* 30 (1974): 864–865.

Burley, N. "The Evolution of Concealed Ovulation." *The American Naturalist* 114 (1979): 835–838.

Cabanac, M. "Physiological Role of Pleasure." *Science* 173 (1971): 1103–1107.

Cain, W. S. "Bilateral Interaction in Olfaction." *Nature* 268 (1977): 50–52.

——— . "Odor Identification by Males and Females: Predictions vs. Performance." *Chemical Senses* 7 (1982): 129–142.

Cain, W. S., and C. L. Murphy. "Interaction between Chemoreceptive Modalities of Odour and Irritation." *Nature* 284 (1980): 255–257.

Cain, W. S., and E. H. Polak. "Olfactory Adaptation as an Aspect of Odor Similarity." *Chemical Senses* 17 (1992): 481–491.

Calvin, W. H. *The River That Flows Uphill*. New York: Macmillan, 1986.

Cann, A., and D. A. Ross. "Olfactory Stimuli as Context Cues in Human Memory." *American Journal of Psychology* 102 (1989): 91–102.

Carr, W. E. S., R. A. Gleeson, and H. G. Trapido-Rosenthal. "The Role of Perireceptor Events in Chemosensory Processes." *Trends in Neurosciences* 13 (1990): 212-215.

Cavalini, P. M. "It's an Ill Wind That Blows No Good: Studies on Odor Annoyance and the Dispersion of Odorant Concentrations from Industries." Ph.D. diss., Rijksuniversiteit Groningen, 1992.

Cernoch, J. M., and R. H. Porter. "Recognition of Maternal Axillary Odors by Infants." *Child Development* 56 (1985): 1593-1598.

Chastrette, M., A. Elmouaffek, and P. Sauvegrain. "A Multidimensional Statistical Study of Similarities between Seventy-four Notes Used in Perfumery." *Chemical Senses* 13 (1988): 295-305.

Chastrette, M., and D. Zakarya. "Molecular Structure and Smell." In *The Human Sense of Smell*, edited by D. G. Laing, R. L. Doty, and W. Breipohl. Berlin: Springer, 1991.

Claassen, J. *Tussen neus en lippen*. Baarn, Netherlands: Tirion, 1993.

Clark, T. "Whose Pheromone Are You?" *World Medicine*, 26 July 1978, 21-23.

Claus, R., and W. Alsing. "Occurrence of 5-α-androst-16-en-3-one, a Boar Pheromone, in Man and Its Relationship to Testosterone." *Journal of Endocrinology* 68 (1976): 483-484.

Claus, R., H. O. Hoppen, and H. Karg. "The Secret of Truffles: A Steroidal Pheromone?" *Experientia* 37 (1981): 1178-1179.

Cometto-Muñiz, J. E., and W. S. Cain. "Thresholds for Odor and Nasal Pungency." *Physiology and Behavior* 48 (1990): 719-725.

Comfort, A. "Likelihood of Human Pheromones." *Nature* 230 (1971): 432-433.

Corbin, A. *Pestdamp en bloesemgeur*. Nijmegen, Netherlands: SUN, 1986.

Costanzo, R. M., and P. P. C. Graziadei. "Development and Plasticity of the Olfactory System." In *Neurobiology of Taste and Smell*, edited by T. E. Finger and W. L. Silver. New York: Wiley, 1987.

Cowley, A. L., A. L. Johnson, and B. W. L. Brooksbank. "The Effect of Two Odorous Compounds in an Assessment-of-People Test." *Psychoneuroendocrinology* 2 (1977): 159-172.

Curtis, R. F., J. A. Ballantine, E. B. Keverne, R. W. Bonsall, and R. P. Michael. "Identification of Primate Sexual Pheromones and the Properties of Synthetic Attractants." *Nature* 232 (1971): 396-398.

Cutler, W. B., G. Preti, G. R. Erickson, G. R. Huggins, and C. R. Garcia. "Sexual Behavior Frequency and Ovulatory Biphasic Menstrual Cycle Patterns." *Physiology and Behavior* 34 (1985): 805-810.

Cutler, W. B., G. Preti, A. Krieger, G. R. Huggins, C. R. Garcia, and H. J. Lawley. "Human Axillary Secretions Influence Women's Menstrual Cycles: The Role of Donor Extract from Men." *Hormones and Behavior* 20 (1986): 463-473.

Davis, R. G., and R. M. Pangborn. "Odor Pleasantness Judgments Compared among Samples from Twenty Nations Using Microfragrances." *Chemical Senses* 10 (1985): 413.

Dawkins, R. *The Extended Phenotype*. Oxford, U.K.: W. H. Freeman, 1982.

Debagge, P. L., N. J. Klein, D. S. O'Dell, D. A. Fraser, and D. W. James. "The Culture of Olfactory Neurons." *Journal of Anatomy* 135 (1982): 816-817.

Deems, D. A., R. L. Doty, R. G. Settle, and J. B. Snow Jr. "Chemosensory Dysfunction: Analysis of 750 Patients from the University of Pennsylvania Smell and Taste Center." *Chemical Senses* 10 (1985): 683.

Delong, R. E., and T. V. Getchell. "Nasal Respiratory Function—Vasomotor and Secretory Regulation." *Chemical Senses* 12 (1987): 3-36.

Doty, R. L. "Influences of Aging on Human Olfactory Function." In *The Human Sense of Smell*, edited by D. G. Laing, R. L. Doty, and W. Breipohl. Berlin: Springer, 1991.

———. "Odor-Guided Behavior in Mammals." *Experientia* 42 (1986): 257-271.

———. "Olfaction." In *Handbook of Neuropsychology*. Vol. 4. Edited by F. Boller and J. Grafman, 213-228. Amsterdam: Elsevier, 1990.

———. "Olfactory Communication in Humans." *Chemical Senses* 6 (1981): 351-376.

———. "Olfactory Function in Neonates." In *The Human Sense of Smell*, edited by D. G. Laing, R. L. Doty, and W. Breipohl. Berlin: Springer, 1991.

———. "Psychophysical Measurement of Odor Perception in Humans." In *The Human Sense of Smell*, edited by D. G. Laing, R. L. Doty, and W. Breipohl. Berlin: Springer, 1991.

Doty, R. L., S. Applebaum, H. Zusho, and R. G. Settle. "Sex Differences in Odor Identification Ability: A Cross-Cultural Analysis." *Neuropsychologia* 23 (1985): 667-672.

Doty, R. L., P. A. Green, C. Ram, and S. L. Yankell. "Communication of Gender from Human Breath Odors: Relationship to Perceived Intensity and Pleasantness." *Hormones and Behavior* 16 (1982): 13-22.

Doty, R. L., P. F. Reyes, and T. Gregor. "Presence of Both Odor Identification and Detection Deficits in Alzheimer's Disease." *Brain Research Bulletin* 18 (1987): 597-600.

Doty, R. L., P. Shaman, S. L. Applebaum, R. Giberson, L. Sikorski, and L. Rosenberg. "Smell Identification Ability: Changes with Age." *Science* 226 (1984): 1441-1443.

Doty, R. L., P. Shaman, and M. Dann. "Development of the University of Pennsylvania Smell Identification Test: A Standardized Microencapsulated Test of Olfactory Function." *Physiology and Behavior* (Monographs) 32 (1984): 489-496.

Doty, R. L., P. J. Snyder, G. R. Huggins, and L. D. Lowry. "Endocrine, Cardiovascular, and Psychological Correlates of Olfactory Sensitivity Changes during the Human Menstrual Cycle." *Journal of Comparative Physiology and Psychology* 95 (1981): 45-51.

Edwards, D. A., R. A. Mather, S. G. Shirley, and G. H. Dodd. "Evidence for an Olfactory Receptor Which Responds to Nicotine—Nicotine as an Odorant." *Experientia* 43 (1987): 868-873.

Ehrlichman, H., and J. N. Halpern. "Affect and Memory: Effects of Pleasant and

Unpleasant Odors on Retrieval of Happy and Unhappy Memories." *Journal of Personality and Social Psychology* 55 (1988): 769-779.

Engen, T. "The Acquisition of Odor Hedonics." In *Perfumery: The Psychology and Biology of Fragrance*, edited by S. van Toller and G. H. Dodd. New York: Chapman and Hall, 1988.

——. *The Perception of Odors*. New York: Academic Press, 1982.

——. "Remembering Odors and Their Names." *American Scientist* 75 (1987): 497-503.

Engstrom, J. E., L. E. Kanin, and M. A. Klein. "Vitamin C Intake and Mortality among a Sample of the United States Population." *Epidemiology* 3 (1992): 194-202.

Enns, M. P., and D. E. Hornung. "Comparisons of the Estimates of Smell, Taste, and Overall Intensity in Young and Elderly People." *Chemical Senses* 13 (1988): 131-139.

——. "Contributions of Smell and Taste to Overall Intensity." *Chemical Senses* 10 (1985): 357-366.

Epple, G. "Primate Pheromones." In *Pheromones*, edited by M. C. Birch. London: North-Holland, 1974.

Eskenazi, B., W. S. Cain, and K. Friend. "Exploration of Olfactory Aptitude." *Bulletin of the Psychonomic Society* 24 (1986): 203-206.

Eslinger, P. J., A. R. Damasio, and G. W. van Hoesen. "Olfactory Dysfunction in Man: Anatomical and Behavioral Aspects." *Brain and Cognition* 1 (1982): 259-285.

Estrum, S. A., and G. Renner. "Disorders of Taste and Smell." *The Otolaryngology Clinics of North America*. Vol. 20, no. 1. Philadelphia: W. B. Saunders, 1987.

Fahy, T. A., P. Desilva, P. Silverstone, and G. F. Russell. "The Effects of Loss of Taste and Smell in a Case of Anorexia Nervosa and Bulimia Nervosa." *British Journal of Psychiatry* 155 (1989): 860-861.

Farbman, A. I. "Olfactory Neurogenesis: Genetic or Environmental Controls?" *Trends in Neurosciences* 13 (1990): 362-365.

Filiatre, J. C., J. L. Millot, and A. Eckerlin. "Behavioural Variability of Olfactory Exploration of the Pet Dog in Relation to Human Adults." *Applied Animal Behaviour Science* 30 (1991): 341-350.

Filsinger, E., and R. A. Fabes. "Odor Communication, Pheromones, and Human Families." *Journal of Marriage and the Family* 47 (1985): 349-359.

Finger, T. E., and W. L. Silver, eds. *Neurobiology of Taste and Smell*. New York: Wiley, 1987.

Freeland, W. J. "Mangabey (*Cercocebus albigena*) Movement Patterns in Relation to Food Availability and Fecal Contamination." *Ecology* 61 (1980): 1297-1303.

Freeman, W. J. "The Physiology of Perception." *Scientific American*, February 1991, 34-41.

Freeman, W. J., and K. A. Grajski. "Relation of Olfactory EEG to Behavior: Factor Analysis." *Behavioral Neuroscience* 101 (1987): 766-777.

Frijda, N. *The Emotions*. Cambridge: Cambridge University Press, 1986.

Frisch, K. von. *Bees: Their Chemical Senses, Vision, and Language.* Ithaca, N.Y.: Cornell University Press, 1950.

Geldard, F. A. *The Human Senses.* New York: Wiley, 1972.

Getchell, T. V., and M. L. Getchell. "Peripheral Mechanisms of Olfaction: Biochemistry and Neurophysiology." In *Neurobiology of Taste and Smell,* edited by T. E. Finger and W. L. Silver. New York: Wiley, 1991.

———. "Physiology of Olfactory Reception and Transduction: General Principles." In *The Human Sense of Smell,* edited by D. G. Laing, R. L. Doty, and W. Breipohl. Berlin: Springer, 1991.

Gibbons, B. "The Intimate Sense of Smell." *National Geographic,* September 1986, 324–360.

Gilbert, A. N., A. J. Fridlund, and J. Sabini. "Hedonic and Social Determinants of Facial Displays to Odors." *Chemical Senses* 12 (1987): 355–363.

Gonzales, F., and A. I. Farbman. "Developing Olfactory Receptor Cells Grow Axons in Tissue Culture." *In Vitro* 20 (1984): 268.

Gould, S. J., and R. C. Lewontin. "The Spandrels of San Marco and the Panglossian Paradigm: A Critique of the Adaptationist Programme." *Proceedings of the Royal Society of London* B205 (1979): 581–598.

Gower, D. B. "Biosynthesis of the Androgens and Other C19 Steroids." In *Biochemistry of Steroid Hormones,* edited by H. L. J. Makin. 2d ed. Oxford, U.K.: Blackwell, 1984.

Gower, D. B., S. Bird, P. Sharma, and F. R. House. "Axillary 5-α-androst-16-en-3-one in Men and Women: Relationships with Olfactory Acuity of Odorous 16-androstenes." *Experientia* 41 (1985): 1134–1136.

Gower, D. B., A. Nixon, and A. I. Mallet. "The Significance of Odorous Steroids in Axillary Odor." In *Perfumery: The Psychology and Biology of Fragrance,* edited by S. van Toller and G. H. Dodd. New York: Chapman and Hall, 1988.

Gross-Isseroff, R., and D. Lancet. "Concentration-Dependent Changes of Perceived Odor Quality." *Chemical Senses* 13 (1988): 191–204.

Gustavson, A. R., M. E. Dawson, and D. G. Bonett. "Androstenol, a Putative Human Pheromone, Affects Human (*Homo sapiens*) Male Choice Performance." *Journal of Comparative Psychology* 101 (1987): 210–212.

Haberly, L. B., and J. M. Bower. "Olfactory Cortex: Model Circuit for Study of Associative Memory?" *Trends in Neurosciences* 12 (1989): 258–264.

Hamilton, W. D. "The Genetical Evolution of Social Behavior." *Journal of Theoretical Biology* 7 (1964): 1–52.

Harrington, A. *Medicine, Mind, and the Double Brain.* Princeton, N.J.: Princeton University Press, 1987.

Harrison, P. J., and R. C. A. Pearson. "Olfaction and Psychiatry." *British Journal of Psychiatry* 155 (1989): 822–828.

Hart, M. 't. *Verzamelde verhalen.* Amsterdam: De Arbeiderspers, 1992.

Hendriks, A. P. J. "Olfactory Dysfunction." *Rhinology* 26 (1988): 229–251.

Henning, H. *Der Geruch.* 2d ed. Leipzig: Barth, 1924.

Hepper, P. G. "The Amniotic Fluid: An Important Priming Role in Kin Recognition." *Animal Behaviour* 35 (1987): 1343-1346.

———. "The Discrimination of Human Odour by the Dog." *Perception* 17 (1988): 549-554.

Herz, R. S., and G. C. Cupchik. "An Experimental Characterization of Odor-Evoked Memories in Humans." *Chemical Senses* 17 (1992): 519-528.

Heukels, H., and S. J. van Ooststroom. *Flora van Nederland*. Groningen: Wolters-Noordhoff, 1977.

Hinde, R. A. "A Conceptual Framework." In *Primate Social Relationships: An Integrated Approach*, edited by R. A. Hinde. Oxford, U.K.: Blackwell, 1983.

Hoes, M. J. A. "Historiografie II: De personae." *Soma en Psyche*, January 1994, 12-33.

Hold, B., and M. Schleidt. "The Importance of Human Odor in Nonverbal Communication." *Zeitschrift für Tierpsychologie* 43 (1977): 225-238.

Hummel, T., R. Gollisch, G. Wildt, and G. Kobal. "Changes in Olfactory Perception during the Menstrual Cycle." *Experientia* 47 (1991): 712-715.

Hvastja, L., and L. Zanuttini. "Odour Memory and Odour Hedonics in Children." *Perception* 18 (1989): 391-396.

Izard, M. K. "Pheromones and Reproduction in Domestic Animals." In *Pheromones and Reproduction in Mammals*, edited by J. G. Vandenbergh. New York: Academic Press, 1983.

Jacobson, M., M. Beroza, and W. A. Jones. "Isolation, Identification, and Synthesis of the Sex Attractant of the Gypsy Moth." *Science* 132 (1960): 1011.

Jansen, A. "Binge Eating." Ph.D. diss., Meppel, Krips Repro, 1990.

Jelicic, M. "Unconscious Auditory Information Processing during General Anesthesia." Ph.D. diss., Erasmusuniversiteit Rotterdam, 1992.

Jerison, H. "The Evolution of Biological Intelligence." In *Handbook of Human Intelligence*, edited by R. J. Sternberd. Cambridge: Cambridge University Press, 1982.

Jessee, J. "The Sense of Smell Awakens Nostalgia." *Dragoco Report* 3 (1982): 76.

Johnston, R. E. "Chemical Signals and Reproductive Behavior." In *Pheromones and Reproduction in Mammals*, edited by J. G. Vandenbergh. New York: Academic Press, 1983.

Karlson, P., and M. Lüscher. "Pheromones: A New Term for a Class of Biologically Active Substances." *Nature* 183 (1959): 55-56.

Katan, M. "Steeds ouder, maar gelukkiger?" Interview by Jan Tromp. *De Volkskrant (Het Vervolg)*, 27 March 1993.

Kauer, J. S. "Coding in the Olfactory System." In *Neurobiology of Taste and Smell*, edited by T. E. Finger and W. L. Silver. New York: Wiley, 1987.

Kay, R. W. "Geomagnetic Storms: Association with Incidence of Depression as Measured by Hospital Admission." *British Journal of Psychiatry* 164 (1994): 403-409.

Kayzer, W. *A Glorious Accident*. Princeton, N.J.: Films for the Humanities and Sciences, 1994.

Keverne, E. B., C. L. Murphy, W. L. Silver, C. J. Wysocki, and M. Meredith. "Nonolfactory Chemoreceptors of the Nose: Recent Advances in Understanding the Vomeronasal and Trigeminal Systems." *Chemical Senses* 11 (1986): 119-133.

King, J. R. "Anxiety Reduction Using Fragrances." In *Perfumery: The Psychology and Biology of Fragrance*, edited by S. van Toller and G. H. Dodd. New York: Chapman and Hall, 1988.

Kirk-Smith, M. D., and D. A. Booth. "Effects of Androstenone on Choice of Location in Others' Presence." In *Olfaction and Taste*. Vol. 7, edited by H. van der Starre. London: IRL Press, 1980.

Kirk-Smith, M. D., D. A. Booth, D. Carroll, and P. Davies. "Human Social Attitudes Affected by Androstenol." *Research Communications in Psychology, Psychiatry, and Behavior* 3 (1978): 379-384.

Kirk-Smith, M. D., S. van Toller, and G. H. Dodd. "Unconscious Odor Conditioning in Human Subjects." *Biological Psychology* 17 (1983): 221-231.

Kneissler, M. "Wir mutieren." *Wiener*, May 1989.

Kobal, G., S. van Toller, and T. Hummel. "Is There Directional Smelling?" *Experientia* 45 (1989): 130-132.

Koelega, H. S. "Preference for and Sensitivity to the Odors of Androstenone and Musk." In *Olfaction and Taste*. Vol. 7, edited by H. van der Starre. London: IRL Press, 1980.

Korsching, S. "Sniffing Out Odorant Receptors." *Trends in Biochemical Sciences* 16 (1991): 277-278.

Köster, E. P. "Adaptation and Cross Adaptation in Olfaction." Ph.D. diss., Rijksuniversiteit Utrecht, 1971.

―――. "De funktie van de reukzin." In *Psychologie in Nederland*, edited by J. C. J. Bonarius, et al. Vol. 2, 1-14. Lisse: Swets en Zeitlinger, 1986.

―――. "Over geur en stank." In *Proeven op de som*, edited by W. A. Wagenaar, P. A. Vroon, and W. H. Janssen. Deventer, Netherlands: Van Loghum Slaterus, 1978.

Köster, E. P., and R. A. de Wijk. "Olfactory Adaptation." In *The Human Sense of Smell*, edited by D. G. Laing, R. L. Doty, and W. Breipohl. Berlin: Springer, 1991.

Kucharski, D., and W. G. Hall. "New Routes to Early Memories. *Science* 238 (1987): 786-788.

La Fontaine, J. S. *The Extent and Nature of Organised and Ritual Abuse*. London: Department of Health, 1994.

Laing, D. G. "Characteristics of the Human Sense of Smell When Processing Odor Mixtures." In *The Human Sense of Smell*, edited by D. G. Laing, R. L. Doty, and W. Breipohl. Berlin: Springer, 1991.

―――. "Identification of Single Dissimilar Odors Is Achieved by Humans with a Single Sniff." *Physiology and Behavior* 37 (1986): 163-170.

Laing, D. G., R. L. Doty, and W. Breipohl, eds. *The Human Sense of Smell*. Berlin: Springer, 1991.

Laing, D. G., and G. W. Francis. "The Capacity of Humans to Identify Odors in Mixtures." *Physiology and Behavior* 46 (1989): 809-814.

Laing, D. G., and A. Glemarec. "Selective Attention and the Perceptual Analysis of Odor Mixtures." *Physiology and Behavior* 52 (1992): 1047-1053.

Laing, D. G., and P. Macleod. "Reaction Time for the Recognition of Odor Quality." *Chemical Senses* 17 (1992): 337-346.

Laing, D. G., and M. E. Willcox. "Perception of Components in Binary Odor Mixtures." *Chemical Senses* 7 (1983): 249-264.

Lancet, D. "Vertebrate Olfactory Reception." *Annual Review of Neurosciences* 9 (1986): 329-355.

Lancet, D., and U. Pace. "The Molecular Basis of Odor Recognition." *Trends in Biochemical Sciences* 12 (1987): 63-66.

Laska, M., and R. Hudson. "Ability to Discriminate between Related Odor Mixtures." *Chemical Senses* 17 (1992): 403-415.

Lawless, H. "Effects of Odors on Mood and Behavior: Aromatherapy and Related Effects." In *The Human Sense of Smell*, edited by D. G. Laing, R. L. Doty, and W. Breipohl. Berlin: Springer, 1991.

Le Gros Clark, W. E. "The Structure of the Brain and the Process of Thinking." In *The Physical Basis of Thinking*, edited by P. Lashlett. Oxford, U.K.: Blackwell, 1952.

Le Magnen, J. "Les Phénomènes olfacto-sexuels chez l'homme." *Archives des Sciences Physiologiques* 6 (1952): 125-160.

Lord, T., and M. Kasprzak. "Identification of Self through Olfaction." *Perceptual and Motor Skills* 69 (1989): 219-224.

Lorenz, K. *Studies in Animal and Human Behavior*. 2 vols. Translated by Robert Martin. Cambridge, Mass.: Harvard University Press, 1970-1971.

Lorig, T. S., and G. E. Schwartz. "Brain and Odor: I. Alteration of Human EEG by Odor Administration." *Psychobiology* 16 (1988): 281-284.

Lorig, T. S., G. E. Schwartz, K. B. Herman, and R. D. Lane. "Brain and Odor: II. EEG Activity during Nose and Mouth Breathing." *Psychobiology* 16 (1988): 285-287.

Ludvigson, H. W., and T. R. Rottman. "Effects of Ambient Odors of Lavender and Cloves on Cognition, Memory, Affect, and Mood." *Chemical Senses* 14 (1989): 525-536.

Lyman, B. J., and M. A. McDaniel. "Effects of Encoding Strategy on Long-Term Memory of Odors." *The Quarterly Journal of Experimental Psychology* 38a (1986): 753-765.

———. "Memory for Odors and Odor Names: Modalities of Elaboration and Imagery." *Journal of Experimental Psychology: Learning, Memory, and Cognition* 16 (1990): 656-664.

Macht, D. I., and G. C. Ting. "Experimental Inquiry into the Sedative Effects of Some Aromatic Drugs and Fumes." *Journal of Pharmacology and Experimental Therapy* 18 (1921): 361-372.

MacLean, P. D. *The Triune Brain in Evolution*. New York: Plenum Press, 1990.

Macrides, F., T. A. Schoenfeld, J. E. Marchand, and A. N. Clancy. "Evidence for Morphologically, Neurochemically, and Functionally Heterogeneous Classes of Mitral and Tufted Cells in the Olfactory Bulb." *Chemical Senses* 10 (1985): 175-202.

Mair, R. G., R. L. Doty, K. M. Kelly, C. S. Wilson, P. J. Langlais, W. J. McEntee, and T. A. Vollmecke. "Multimodal Sensory Discrimination Deficits in Korsakoff's Psychosis." *Neuropsychologia* 24 (1986): 831-839.

Mair, R. G., and L. M. Harrison. "Influence of Drugs on Smell Function." In *The Human Sense of Smell*, edited by D. G. Laing, R. L. Doty, and W. Breipohl. Berlin: Springer, 1991.

Margolis, F. L. "Olfactory Marker Protein: From Page Band to CDNA Clone." *Trends in Neurosciences* 8 (1985): 542-546.

Marks, L. E., J. C. Stevens, L. M. Bartoshuk, J. F. Gent, B. Rifkin, and V. K. Stone. "Magnitude-Matching: The Measurement of Taste and Smell." *Chemical Senses* 13 (1988): 63-87.

Mason, J. R., L. Clark, and T. H. Morton. "Selective Deficits in the Sense of Smell Caused by Chemical Modification of the Olfactory Epithelium." *Science* 226 (1984): 1092-1094.

McClintock, M. K. "Menstrual Synchrony and Suppression." *Nature* 229 (1971): 244-245.

———. "Pheromonal Regulation of the Ovarian Cycle: Enhancement, Suppression, and Synchrony." In *Pheromones and Reproduction in Mammals*, edited by J. G. Vandenbergh. New York: Academic Press, 1983.

McCollough, P. A., J. W. Owen, and E. I. Pollak. "Does Androstenol Affect Emotion?" *Ethology and Sociobiology* 2 (1981): 85-88.

Melrose, D. R., H. C. B. Reed, and R. L. S. Patterson. "Androgen Steroids as an Aid to the Detection of Oestrus in Pig Artificial Insemination." *British Veterinary Journal* 130 (1974): 61-67.

Mennella, J. A., and G. K. Beauchamp. "Olfactory Preferences in Children and Adults." In *The Human Sense of Smell*, edited by D. G. Laing, R. L. Doty, and W. Breipohl. Berlin: Springer, 1991.

Meredith, M. "Sensory Physiology of Pheromone Communication." In *Pheromones and Reproduction in Mammals*, edited by J. G. Vandenbergh. New York: Academic Press, 1983.

Michael, R. P., R. W. Bonsall, and P. Warner. "Human Vaginal Secretions: Volatile Fatty Acid Contents." *Science* 186 (1974): 1217-1219.

Michael, R. P., J. Herbert, and G. Saayman. "Loss of Ejaculation in Male Rhesus Monkeys after Administration of Progesterone to Their Female Partners: Preliminary Communication." *Lancet* 1 (1966): 1015-1016.

Michael, R. P., and E. B. Keverne. "Pheromones in the Communication of Sexual Status in Primates." *Nature* 218 (1968): 746-749.

Michael, R. P., E. B. Keverne, and R. W. Bonsall. "Pheromones: Isolation of Male Sex Attractants from a Female Primate." *Science* 172 (1971): 964-965.

Millot, J. L., J. C. Filiatre, A. Eckerlin, A. C. Gagnon, and H. Montagner. "Olfactory Cues in the Relations between Children and Their Pet Dogs." *Applied Animal Behaviour Science* 19 (1987): 189-195.

Moir, A., and D. Jessel. *Brain Sex: The Real Difference between Men and Women*. London: M. Joseph, 1989.

Moran, D. T., B. W. Jafek, and J. C. Rowley III. "The Ultrastructure of the Human Olfactory Mucosa." In *The Human Sense of Smell*, edited by D. G. Laing, R. L. Doty, and W. Breipohl. Berlin: Springer, 1991.

Morgan, E. *The Scars of Evolution: What Our Bodies Tell Us About Human Origins*. London: Souvenir Press, 1990.

Morrison, E. E., and P. P. C. Graziadei. "Transplants of Olfactory Mucosa in the Rat Brain, I: A Light Microscopic Study of Transplant Organization." *Brain Research* 279 (1983): 241-245.

Mozell, M. M. "The Chemical Senses, II: Olfaction." In *Woodworth and Schlosberg's Experimental Psychology*, edited by J. W. Kling and L. A. Riggs. 3d ed. New York: Holt, Rinehart and Winston, 1971.

Mozell, M. M., B. P. Smith, P. E. Smith, R. J. Sullivan Jr., and P. Swender. "Nasal Chemoreception and Flavor Identification." *Archives of Otolaryngology* 90 (1969): 131-137.

Murphy, C. "Olfactory Psychophysics." In *Neurobiology of Taste and Smell*, edited by T. E. Finger and W. L. Silver. New York: Wiley, 1987.

Murphy, C., and W. S. Cain. "Odor Identification: The Blind Are Better." *Physiology and Behavior* 37 (1986): 177-180.

Nisbett, R., and L. Ross. *Human Inference*. Englewood Cliffs, N.J.: Prentice-Hall, 1980.

O'Connell, R. J., D. A. Stevens, R. P. Akers, D. M. Coppola, and A. J. Grant. "Individual Differences in the Quantitative and Qualitative Responses of Human Subjects to Various Odors." *Chemical Senses* 14 (1989): 293-302.

Ohloff, G. "Chemistry of Odor Stimuli." *Experientia* 24 (1986): 271-279.

Ornstein, R., and P. Ehrlich. *New World New Mind*. New York: Doubleday, 1989.

Overbosch, P. "A Theoretical Model for the Perceived Intensity in Human Taste and Smell as a Function of Time." *Chemical Senses* 11 (1986): 315-329.

Pace, U., E. Hanski, Y. Salomon, and D. Lancet. "Odorant-Sensitive Adenylate Cyclase May Mediate Olfactory Reception." *Nature* 316 (1985): 255-258.

Pearson, R. C. A., M. M. Esiri, R. W. Hiorns, G. K. Wilcock, and T. P. S. Powell. "Anatomical Correlates of the Distribution of the Pathological Changes in the Neocortex in Alzheimer's Disease." *Proceedings of the National Academy of Science USA* 82 (1985): 4531-4534.

Perl, E., U. Shay, R. Hamburger, and J. E. Steiner. "Taste- and Odor-Reactivity in Elderly Demented Patients." *Chemical Senses* 17 (1992): 779-794.

Pike, L. M., M. P. Enns, and D. E. Hornung. "Quality and Intensity Differences of Carvone Enantiomers When Tested Separately and in Mixtures." *Chemical Senses* 13 (1988): 307-309.

Porter, R. H., R. D. Balogh, J. M. Cernoch, and C. Franchi. "Recognition of Kin through Characteristic Body Odors." *Chemical Senses* 11 (1986): 389-395.

Porter, R. H., J. M. Cernoch, and R. D. Balogh. "Odor Signatures and Kin Recognition." *Physiology and Behavior* 34 (1985): 445-448.

Porter, R. H., J. M. Cernoch, and F. J. McLaughlin. "Maternal Recognition of Neonates Through Olfactory Cues." *Physiology and Behavior* 30 (1983): 151-154.

Preti, G., W. B. Cutler, G. R. Huggins, C. R. Garcia, and H. J. Lawley. "Human Axillary Secretions Influence Women's Menstrual Cycles: The Role of Donor Extract from Women." *Hormones and Behavior* 20 (1986): 474-482.

Price, J. L. "Beyond the Primary Olfactory Cortex: Olfactory-Related Areas in the Neocortex, Thalamus, and Hypothalamus." *Chemical Senses* 10 (1985): 239-258.

———. "The Central Olfactory and Accessory Olfactory Systems." In *Neurobiology of Taste and Smell*, edited by T. E. Finger and W. L. Silver. New York: Wiley, 1987.

Price, S. "Mechanisms of Stimulation of Olfactory Neurons: An Essay." *Chemical Senses* 8 (1984): 341-354.

Raaijmakers, J. G. W. "De psycholoog als ingenieur." Paper delivered at the Universiteit van Amsterdam, 1993.

Rabin, M. D. "Experience Facilitates Olfactory Quality Discrimination." *Perception and Psychophysics* 44 (1988): 532-540.

Rabin, M. D., and W. S. Cain. "Determinants of Measured Olfactory Sensitivity." *Perception and Psychophysics* 39 (1986): 281-286.

———. "Odor Recognition: Familiarity, Identifiability, and Encoding Consistency." *Journal of Experimental Psychology: Learning, Memory, and Cognition* 10 (1984): 316-325.

Richardson, J. T. E., and G. M. Zucco. "Cognition and Olfaction: A Review." *Psychological Bulletin* 105 (1989): 352-360.

Rindisbacher, H. J. *The Smell of Books: A Cultural-Historical Study of Olfactory Perception in Literature*. Ann Arbor: University of Michigan Press, 1993.

Roede, M., J. Wind, J. Patrick, and V. Reynolds, eds. *The Aquatic Ape: Fact or Fiction?* London: Souvenir Press, 1991.

Rubin, D. C., E. Groth, and D. J. Goldsmith. "Olfactory Cuing of Autobiographical Memory." *American Journal of Psychology* 97 (1984): 493-507.

Russell, M. J. "Human Olfactory Communication." In *Chemical Signals in Vertebrates*, edited by D. Müller-Schwarze and R. Silverstein. Vol. 3. New York: Plenum, 1983.

Russell, M. J., T. Mendelson, and H. V. S. Peeke. "Mothers' Identification of Their Infants' Odors." *Ethology and Sociobiology* 4 (1983): 29-31.

Sacks, O. *The Man Who Mistook His Wife for a Hat*. London: Duckworth, 1985.

Schaal, B. "Olfaction in Infants and Children: Developmental and Functional Perspectives." *Chemical Senses* 13 (1988): 145-190.

Schaal, B., E. Montagner, E. Hertling, D. Bolzini, A. Moyse, and R. Quichon. "Les

Stimulations olfactives dans les relations entre l'enfant et la mère." *Reproduction, Nutrition, Développement* 20, no. 3b (1980): 843–858.

Schab, F. R. "Odor Memory: Taking Stock." *Psychological Bulletin* 109 (1991): 242–251.

———. "Odors and the Remembrance of Things Past." *Journal of Experimental Psychology: Learning, Memory, and Cognition* 16 (1990): 648–655.

Schab, F. R., and W. S. Cain. "Memory for Odors." In *The Human Sense of Smell*, edited by D. G. Laing, R. L. Doty, and W. Breipohl. Berlin: Springer, 1991.

Schiet, F. T., and J. E. R. Frijters. "An Investigation of the Equiratio-Mixture Model in Olfactory Psychophysics: A Case Study." *Perception and Psychophysics* 44 (1988): 304–308.

Schiffmann, S. "Food Recognition by the Elderly." *Journal of Gerontology* 32 (1977): 586–592.

Schleidt, M., P. Neumann, and H. Morishita. "Pleasure and Disgust: Memories and Associations of Pleasant and Unpleasant Odors in Germany and Japan." *Chemical Senses* 13 (1988): 279–293.

Schmidt, H. J., and G. K. Beauchamp. "Adult-like Odor Preferences and Aversions in Three-Year-Old Children." *Child Development* 59 (1988): 1136–1143.

Schneider, P. "Insect Olfaction: Deciphering System for Chemical Messages." *Science* 163 (1969): 1031–1036.

Schwartz, B. S. "Epidemiology and Its Application to Olfactory Dysfunction." In *The Human Sense of Smell*, edited by D. G. Laing, R. L. Doty, and W. Breipohl. Berlin: Springer, 1991.

Scott, J. W., and T. A. Harrison. "The Olfactory Bulb: Anatomy and Physiology." In *Neurobiology of Taste and Smell*, edited by T. E. Finger and W. L. Silver. New York: Wiley, 1987.

Sheldrake, R. *Seven Experiments That Could Change the World*. London: Fourth Estate, 1994.

Shipley, M. T. "Transport of Molecules from Nose to Brain: Transneuronal Anterograde and Retrograde Labeling in the Rat Olfactory System by Wheat Germ Agglutinin Horseradish to the Nasal Epithelium." *Brain Research Bulletin* 15 (1985): 129–142.

Shipley, M., and P. Reyes. "Anatomy of the Human Olfactory Bulb and Central Olfactory Pathways." In *The Human Sense of Smell*, edited by D. G. Laing, R. L. Doty, and W. Breipohl. Berlin: Springer, 1991.

Sicard, G., and A. Holley. "Receptor Cell Responses to Odorants: Similarities and Differences among Odorants." *Brain Research* 292 (1984): 283–296.

Silver, W. L. "The Common Chemical Sense." In *Neurobiology of Taste and Smell*, edited by T. E. Finger and W. L. Silver. New York: Wiley, 1987.

Simerly, R. B. "Hormonal Control of Neuropeptide Gene Expression in Sexually Dimorphic Olfactory Pathways." *Trends in Neurosciences* 13 (1990): 104–110.

Slotnick, B. M., and A. J. Pazos. "Rats with One Olfactory Bulb Removed and the Contralateral Naris Closed Can Detect Odors." *Physiology and Behavior* 48 (1990): 37-40.

Smith, D. G., L. Standing, and A. de Man. "Verbal Memory Elicited by Ambient Odor." *Perceptual and Motor Skills* 74 (1992): 339-343.

Smith, D. V., and A. M. Seiden. "Olfactory Dysfunction." In *The Human Sense of Smell*, edited by D. G. Laing, R. L. Doty, and W. Breipohl. Berlin: Springer, 1991.

Snyder, S. H. "Opiate Receptors and Internal Opiates." *Scientific American* 236 (1977): 44-56.

Snyder, S. H., P. B. Sklar, P. M. Hwang, and J. Pevsner. "Molecular Mechanisms of Olfaction." *Trends in Neurosciences* 12 (1989): 35-38.

Snyder, S. H., P. B. Sklar, and J. Pevsner. "Molecular Mechanisms of Olfaction." *The Journal of Biological Chemistry* 263 (1988): 13971-13974.

Spaink, K. *Het strafbare lichaam.* Amsterdam: Mutinga, 1992.

Stahlbaum, C. C., and K. A. Houpt. "The Role of the Flehmen Response in the Behavioral Repertoire of the Stallion." *Physiology and Behavior* 45 (1989): 1207-1214.

Stamp Dawkins, M. *Through Our Eyes Only?* Oxford, U.K.: Freeman, 1993.

Staubli, U., D. Fraser, R. Faraday, and G. Lynch. "Olfaction and the 'Data' Memory System in Rats." *Behavioral Neuroscience* 101 (1987): 757-765.

Stevens, J. C., and W. S. Cain. "Age-Related Deficiency in the Perceived Strength of Six Odorants." *Chemical Senses* 10 (1985): 517-529.

———. "Smelling via the Mouth: Effect of Aging." *Perception and Psychophysics* 40 (1986): 142-146.

Stevens, J. C., W. S. Cain, and R. J. Burke. "Variability of Olfactory Thresholds." *Chemical Senses* 13 (1988): 643-653.

Stevens, J. C., W. S. Cain, and A. Demarque. "Memory and Identification of Simulated Odors in Elderly and Young Persons." *Bulletin of the Psychonomic Society* 28 (1990): 293-296.

Stevens, J. C., W. S. Cain, F. T. Schiet, and M. W. Oatley. "Olfactory Adaptation and Recovery in Old Age." *Perception* 18 (1989): 265-276.

Stoddart, D. M. "Human Odor Culture: A Zoological Perspective." In *Perfumery: The Psychology and Biology of Fragrance*, edited by S. van Toller and G. H. Dodd. New York: Chapman and Hall, 1988.

———. *The Scented Ape: The Biology and Culture of Human Odour.* Rev. ed. Cambridge: Cambridge University Press, 1991.

Stuiver, M. "Biophysics of the Sense of Smell." Ph.D. diss., Rijksuniversiteit Groningen, 1958.

Süskind, P. *Perfume: The Story of a Murderer.* Translated by John E. Woods. New York: Alfred A. Knopf, 1986.

Teicher, M. H., and E. M. Blass. "First Suckling Response of the Newborn Albino Rat: The Roles of Olfaction and Amniotic Fluid." *Science* 198 (1977): 635-636.

Tinbergen, N. *Social Behavior in Animals, with Special Reference to Vertebrates.* London: Chapman and Hall, 1990.

Tisserand, R. *Aromatherapy.* London: Penguin, 1988.

Toller, S. van. "Emotion and the Brain." In *Perfumery: The Psychology and Biology of Fragrance,* edited by S. van Toller and G. H. Dodd. New York: Chapman and Hall, 1988.

Toller, S. van, and G. H. Dodd, eds. *Perfumery: The Psychology and Biology of Fragrance.* New York: Chapman and Hall, 1988.

Toller, S. van, G. H. Dodd, and A. Billing, eds. *Aging and the Sense of Smell.* Springfield, Ill., Thomas, 1985.

Toller, S. van, M. Kirk-Smith, N. Wood, J. Lombard, and G. H. Dodd. "Skin-Conductance and Subjective Assessments Associated with the Odour of 5-α-androstan-3-one." *Biological Psychology* 16 (1983): 85–107.

Tuiten, A. "Interactions between Mental and Bodily Mechanisms in Anorexia Nervosa and Premenstrual Complaints." Ph.D. diss., Rijksuniversiteit Utrecht, 1993.

Turke, P. W. "Effects of Ovulatory Concealment and Synchrony on Protohominid Mating Systems and Parental Roles." *Ethology and Sociobiology* 5 (1984): 33–44.

Vandenbergh, J. G., ed. *Pheromones and Reproduction in Mammals.* New York: Academic Press, 1983.

Veith, J., M. Buck, S. Gertzlaf, P. van Dolfsen, and A. Slade. "Exposure to Men Influences the Occurrence of Ovulation in Women." *Physiology and Behavior* 31 (1983): 313–315.

Vroon, P. *Kopzorgen.* Baarn, Netherlands: Ambo, 1990.

———. *Psychologische aspecten van ziekmakende gebouwen.* Utrecht: ISOR, 1990.

———. *Toestanden.* Baarn, Netherlands: Ambo, 1993.

———. *Tranen van de krokodil.* Baarn, Netherlands: Ambo, 1989; published in German as *Drei Hirne im Kopf.* Stuttgart: Kreuz Verlag, 1993.

———. *Wolfskiem.* Baarn, Netherlands: Ambo, 1992.

Vroon, P., and D. Draaisma. *De mens als metafoor.* Baarn, Netherlands: Ambo, 1986.

Walk, H. A., and E. E. Johns. "Interference and Facilitation in Short-Term Memory for Odors." *Perception and Psychophysics* 36 (1984): 508–514.

Wallraff, H. G. "Conceptual Approaches to Avian Navigation Systems." *Experientia* 46 (1990): 379–388.

Warren, D. W., J. C. Walker, A. F. Drake, and R. W. Lutz. "Assessing the Effects of Odorants on Nasal Airway Size and Breathing." *Physiology and Behavior* 51 (1992): 425–430.

Whitten, W. K., F. H. Bronson, and J. A. Greenstein. "Estrus-Inducing Pheromone of Mice: Transport by Movement of Air." *Science* 161 (1968): 584–585.

Williams, M. B. "The Logical Structure of Functional Explanations in Biology." In

PSA 1976: Proceedings of the 1976 Biennial Meeting of the Philosophy of Science Association, edited by F. Suppe and P. D. Asquith, 37–46. East Lansing, Mich.: Philosophy of Science Association, 1976.

Wilson, E. O., and W. H. Bossert. "Chemical Communication among Animals." In *Recent Progress in Hormone Research*, edited by G. Pincus. Vol. 19. New York: Academic Press, 1963.

Wysocki, C. J., and G. K. Beauchamp. "Ability to Smell Androstenone Is Genetically Determined." *Proceedings of the National Academy of Science USA* 81 (1984): 4899–4902.

Wysocki, C. J., and M. Meredith. "The Vomeronasal System." In *Neurobiology of Taste and Smell*, edited by T. E. Finger and W. L. Silver. New York: Wiley, 1987.

Zellner, D. A., and M. A. Kautz. "Color Affects Perceived Odor Intensity." *Journal of Experimental Psychology: Human Perception and Performance* 16 (1990): 391–397.

Zwaan, E. J. "Links en rechts in waarneming en beleving." Ph.D. diss., Utrecht: Bijleveld, 1965.